CONTENTS

		PAGE
	Preface	2
	Age-Per-Page guidelines	3
ARREST	Paediatric Cardiac Arrest Algorithm	20
	Newborn Cardiac Arrest Algorithm	21
	Peri-Arrest Algorithms	
	Bradycardia	22
	SVT	23
	VT	24
	Peri-Arrest Drugs	25
	Treatment of Hyperkalaemia	26
TRAUMA	Massive Haemorrhage	27
	Traumatic Brain Injury	28
	Children's GCS	28
	Burns	30
	Radiology Guidelines	31
ANAESTHETIC	Difficult Mask Ventilation	33
	Unanticipated Difficult Intubation	34
	Can't Intubate, Can't Ventilate	35
	Malignant Hyperthermia	36
	IV Dantrolene dosing	37
	Severe Local Anaesthetic Toxicity	38
	IV Intralipid dosing	39
	Pain Management Guidelines	40
	Antiemetics	41
	Fluid Management	42
	Congenital Cardiac Disease	44
	CCD for Non-Cardiac Surgery	45
	Common Syndromes & Congenital Conditions	46
MEDICAL	Anaphylaxis	54
	Airway Emergencies	55
	Septic Shock	56
	Status Epilepticus	57
	Life-threatening Asthma	58
	Diabetic Ketoacidosis	59
	DKA associated Cerebral Oedema	60
	Formulary	61
	Steroid replacement therapy	62
	Notes	65
	References	66

PREFACE

Anaesthetising children can be daunting for the trainee or non-specialist Consultant Anaesthetist. The management of paediatric emergencies requires the rapid recall of multiple formulae, drug doses and management guidelines for a multitude of clinical conditions. To provide evidence-based care, clinicians require rapid access to national guidelines presented in a format that enables easy comprehension and application to the clinical scenario.

This book began as a compilation of local treatment guidelines, collated for our anaesthetic trainees. It quickly grew as new sections were added, becoming, we feel, a comprehensive companion for dealing with paediatric emergencies. The aim of the book is to allow confident patient management by non-specialist clinicians in stressful situations without needing to remember formulae, reducing potentially harmful errors.

The book is a collection of 23 flow chart management plans for life-threatening paediatric crises. Topics included in the emergency management guidelines section are:-

- Cardio-pulmonary arrest – Including management of peri-arrest arrhythmia.
- Trauma – Traumatic head injury, massive haemorrhage and burns.
- Anaesthesia – Airway management algorithms, malignant hyperpyrexia, local anaesthetic toxicity, analgesia and fluid management, anaesthetic implications of 50 common conditions and syndromes.
- Medicine – Anaphylaxis, asthma, status epilepticus, sepsis and diabetic ketoacidosis.

The 'age-by-page' section provides pre-calculated drug doses and equipment selections fo children from birth to 12 years, ensuring rapid data access and reducing potentially harmfu errors.

This is not a textbook of paediatric anaesthesia. It is a comprehensive compendium covering the management of a wide range of paediatric emergencies which provides a succinct summary o management plans for trainees in many paediatric specialties.

We would like to acknowledge the contributions made by three anaesthetic trainees (Joy Abbott, Helen Fenner and Katherine James) to the original local guidelines book and also to Andrew Wignell (Paediatric pharmacist) who has checked all of the medication doses used and our calculations.

AGE : TERM

Wt: 3 – 3.5 kg	HR: 110 – 160	RR: 30 – 40	Systolic BP: 70 – 80

AIRWAY

OP Airway: Size: 000	ET Tube:		2.5 – 3.0
	Diameter:	Cuffed:	3.0 – 3.5
LMA: Size: 1		Uncuffed:	9 – 10 cm
	Length (Oral):		

CARDIAC

Defibrillation (4 J/kg)	20 J	Adrenaline	IV – Arrest (10 microgram/kg)	0.4 mL (1 in 10,000)
Atropine (20 microgram/kg)	100 microgram (min)		IM – Anaphylaxis (10 microgram/kg)	0.4 mL (1 in 10,000)
Amiodarone (5 mg/kg)	18 mg (0.6 mL of minijet)		Nebulised – Croup (400 microgram/kg)	1.4 mL (1 in 1,000)

FLUIDS

Crystalloids :	Trauma (10 mL/kg): Other (20 mL/kg) :	35 mL 70 mL	Blood, FFP or Platelets (10 mL/kg)	35 mL
10% Dextrose : (Hypoglycaemia) (2 mL/kg)		7 mL	Mannitol 20% (0.25 – 0.5 g/kg)	4 – 8 mL (0.5 g/kg = 2.5 mL/kg)

DRUGS

Drug (Dose)	Neat or Dilution (mg/mL)	Calculated Dose (3.5 kg)	Volume to be given (mL)
Propofol (1 – 4 mg/kg)	NEAT (10 mg/mL)	3 – 15 mg	0.3 – 1.5 mL
Ketamine IV (2 mg/kg)	NEAT (10 mg/mL)	7 mg	0.7 mL
Fentanyl (1 – 2 microgram/kg)	Dilute to 10 microgram/mL	4 - 7 microgram	0.4 – 0.7 mL
Morphine (0.1 mg/kg)	Dilute to 1 mg/mL	0.3 mg (Repeat PRN)	0.3 mL
Paracetamol IV (10 mg/kg)	NEAT (10 mg/mL)	35 mg	3.5 mL
Suxamethonium (2 mg/kg)	Dilute to 10 mg/mL	7 mg	0.7 mL
Rocuronium (1 mg/kg)	NEAT (10 mg/mL)	3.5 mg	0.35 mL
Atracurium (0.5 mg/kg)	NEAT (10 mg/mL)	2 mg	0.2 mL
Sugammadex (16 mg/kg)	NEAT (100 mg/mL)	50 mg	0.5 mL
Tranexamic Acid (15 mg/kg)	NEAT (100 mg/mL)	50 mg	0.5 mL
10% Calcium Chloride (0.2 mL/kg)	NEAT	0.7 mL	0.7 mL

INFUSIONS

Drug	To Make Up in 50 mL	Infusion Rate
Propofol (4 – 12 mg/kg/hr)	NEAT (10 mg/mL)	2 – 6 mL/hr
Morphine (10 – 40 microgram/kg/hr)	3.5 mg (1 mg/kg)	0.5 – 2 mL/hr (1 mL/hr = 20 microgram/kg/hr)
Midazolam (60 – 240 microgram/kg/hr)	21 mg (6 mg/kg)	0.5 – 2 mL/hr (1 mL/hr = 120 microgram/kg/hr)
Noradrenaline / Adrenaline (0.01 – 0.5 microgram/kg/min)	1 mg (0.3 mg/kg) in 5% Dextrose	0.1 – 5 mL/hr (1 mL/hr = 0.1 microgram/kg/min)

AGE : 3 months

Wt :	4 – 6 kg	HR :	110 – 160	RR :	30 – 40	Systolic BP :	70 – 80

AIRWAY

OP Airway :	Size : 00	ET Tube : Diameter :	Cuffed:	2.5 – 3.0
			Uncuffed:	3.0 – 3.5
LMA :	Size : 1	Length (Oral) :		11 cm

CARDIAC

Defibrillation (4 J/kg)	20 J		IV – Arrest (10 microgram/kg)	0.5 mL (1 in 10,000)
Atropine (20 microgram/kg)	110 microgram	Adrenaline	IM – Anaphylaxis (10 microgram/kg)	0.5 mL (1 in 10,000)
Amiodarone (5 mg/kg)	28 mg (0.6 mL of minijet)		Nebulised – Croup (400 microgram/kg)	2.2 mL (1 in 1,000)

FLUIDS

Crystalloids :	Trauma (10 mL/kg): Other (20 mL/kg) :	55 mL 110 mL	Blood, FFP or Platelets (10 mL/kg)	55 mL
10% Dextrose : (Hypoglycaemia) (2 mL/kg)		12 mL	Mannitol 20% (0.25 – 0.5 g/kg)	7 – 14 mL (0.5 g/kg = 2.5 mL/kg)

DRUGS

Drug (Dose)	Neat or Dilution (mg/mL)	Calculated Dose (5.5 kg)	Volume to be given (mL)
Propofol (1 – 4 mg/kg)	NEAT (10 mg/mL)	5 – 20 mg	0.5 – 2 mL
Ketamine IV (2 mg/kg)	NEAT (10 mg/mL)	10 mg	1 mL
Fentanyl (1 – 2 microgram/kg)	Dilute to 10 microgram/mL	5 – 10 microgram	0.5 – 1 mL
Morphine (0.1 mg/kg)	Dilute to 1 mg/mL	0.5 mg (Repeat PRN)	0.5 mL
Paracetamol IV (15 mg/kg)	NEAT (10 mg/mL)	80 mg	8 mL
Suxamethonium (2 mg/kg)	Dilute to 10 mg/mL	10 mg	1 mL
Rocuronium (1 mg/kg)	NEAT (10 mg/mL)	5 mg	0.5 mL
Atracurium (0.5 mg/kg)	NEAT (10 mg/mL)	2.5 mg	0.25 mL
Sugammadex (16 mg/kg)	NEAT (100 mg/mL)	90 mg	0.9 mL
Tranexamic Acid (15 mg/kg)	NEAT (100 mg/mL)	80 mg	0.8 mL
10% Calcium Chloride (0.2 mL/kg)	NEAT	1.1 mL	1.1 mL

INFUSIONS

Drug	To Make Up in 50 mL	Infusion Rate
Propofol (4 – 12 mg/kg/hr)	NEAT (10 mg/mL)	2 – 6 mL/hr
Morphine (10 – 40 microgram/kg/hr)	5.5 mg (1 mg/kg)	0.5 – 2 mL/hr (1 mL/hr = 20 microgram/kg/hr)
Midazolam (60 – 240 microgram/kg/hr)	30 mg (6 mg/kg)	0.5 – 2 mL/hr (1 mL/hr = 120 microgram/kg/hr)
Noradrenaline / Adrenaline (0.01 – 0.5 microgram/kg/min)	1.5 mg (0.3 mg/kg) in 5% Dextrose	0.1 – 5 mL/hr (1 mL/hr = 0.1 microgram/kg/min)

AGE : 6 months

Wt :	6 – 8 kg	HR :	110 – 160	RR :	30 – 40	Systolic BP :	70 – 90

AIRWAY

OP Airway :	Size : 000	ET Tube : Diameter :	Cuffed:	3.0
			Uncuffed:	3.5
LMA :	Size : 1.5	Length (Oral) :		12 cm

CARDIAC

Defibrillation (4 J/kg)	30 J	Adrenaline	IV – Arrest (10 microgram/kg)	0.7 mL (1 in 10,000)
Atropine (20 microgram/kg)	140 microgram		IM – Anaphylaxis (10 microgram/kg)	0.7 mL (1 in 10,000)
Amiodarone (5 mg/kg)	35 mg (1.2 mL of minijet)		Nebulised – Croup (400 microgram/kg)	2.8 mL (1 in 1,000)

FLUIDS

Crystalloids :	Trauma (10 mL/kg): Other (20 mL/kg) :	70 mL 140 mL	Blood, FFP or Platelets (10 mL/kg)	70 mL
10% Dextrose : (Hypoglycaemia) (2 mL/kg)		14 mL	Mannitol 20% (0.25 – 0.5 g/kg)	9 – 18 mL (0.5 g/kg = 2.5 mL/kg)

DRUGS

Drug (Dose)	Neat or Dilution (mg/mL)	Calculated Dose (7 kg)	Volume to be given (mL)
Propofol (1 – 4 mg/kg)	NEAT (10 mg/mL)	7 – 30 mg	0.7 – 3 mL
Ketamine IV (2 mg/kg)	NEAT (10 mg/mL)	15 mg	1.5 mL
Fentanyl (1 – 2 microgram/kg)	Dilute to 10 microgram/mL	7 – 15 microgram	0.7 – 1.5 mL
Morphine (0.1 mg/kg)	Dilute to 1 mg/mL	0.7 mg (Repeat PRN)	0.7 mL
Paracetamol IV (15 mg/kg)	NEAT (10 mg/mL)	100 mg	10 mL
Suxamethonium (2 mg/kg)	Dilute to 10 mg/mL	14 mg	1.4 mL
Rocuronium (1 mg/kg)	NEAT (10 mg/mL)	7 mg	0.7 mL
Atracurium (0.5 mg/kg)	NEAT (10 mg/mL)	4 mg	0.4 mL
Sugammadex (16 mg/kg)	NEAT (100 mg/mL)	120 mg	1.2 mL
Tranexamic Acid (15 mg/kg)	NEAT (100 mg/mL)	100 mg	1 mL
10% Calcium Chloride (0.2 mL/kg)	NEAT	1.4 mL	1.4 mL

INFUSIONS

Drug	To Make Up in 50 mL	Infusion Rate
Propofol (4 – 12 mg/kg/hr)	NEAT (10 mg/mL)	3 – 8 mL/hr
Morphine (10 – 40 microgram/kg/hr)	7 mg (1 mg/kg)	0.5 – 2 mL/hr (1 mL/hr = 20 microgram/kg/hr)
Midazolam (60 – 240 microgram/kg/hr)	42 mg (6 mg/kg)	0.5 – 2 mL/hr (1 mL/hr = 120 microgram/kg/hr)
Noradrenaline / Adrenaline (0.01 – 0.5 microgram/kg/min)	2 mg (0.3 mg/kg) in 5% Dextrose	0.1 – 5 mL/hr (1 mL/hr = 0.1 microgram/kg/min)

AGE : 9 months

Wt : 7 – 9 kg	HR : 110 – 160	RR : 30 – 40	Systolic BP : 70 – 90

AIRWAY

OP Airway : Size : 00	ET Tube :	3.5
	Diameter : Cuffed:	3.5 – 4.0
LMA : Size : 1.5	Uncuffed: Length (Oral) :	12 cm

CARDIAC

Defibrillation (4 J/kg)	30 J	Adrenaline	IV – Arrest (10 microgram/kg)	0.8 mL (1 in 10,000)
Atropine (20 microgram/kg)	170 microgram		IM – Anaphylaxis (10 microgram/kg)	0.8 mL (1 in 10,000)
Amiodarone (5 mg/kg)	43 mg (1.4 mL of minijet)		Nebulised – Croup (400 microgram/kg)	3.4 mL (1 in 1,000)

FLUIDS

Crystalloids :	Trauma (10 mL/kg): 85 mL	Blood, FFP or	85 mL
	Other (20 mL/kg) : 170 mL	Platelets (10 mL/kg)	
10% Dextrose : (Hypoglycaemia) (2 mL/kg)	17 mL	Mannitol 20% (0.25 – 0.5 g/kg)	10 – 20 mL (0.5 g/kg = 2.5 mL/kg)

DRUGS

Drug (Dose)	Neat or Dilution (mg/mL)	Calculated Dose (8.5 kg)	Volume to be given (mL)
Propofol (1 – 4 mg/kg)	NEAT (10 mg/mL)	8.5 – 35 mg	1 – 3.5 mL
Ketamine IV (2 mg/kg)	NEAT (10 mg/mL)	17 mg	1.7 mL
Fentanyl (1 – 2 microgram/kg)	Dilute to 10 microgram/mL	10 – 20 microgram	1 – 2 mL
Morphine (0.1 mg/kg)	Dilute to 1 mg/mL	0.8 mg (Repeat PRN)	0.8 mL
Paracetamol IV (15 mg/kg)	NEAT (10 mg/mL)	120 mg	12 mL
Suxamethonium (2 mg/kg)	Dilute to 10 mg/mL	17 mg	1.7 mL
Rocuronium (1 mg/kg)	NEAT (10 mg/mL)	8 mg	0.8 mL
Atracurium (0.5 mg/kg)	NEAT (10 mg/mL)	4 mg	0.4 mL
Sugammadex (16 mg/kg)	NEAT (100 mg/mL)	130 mg	1.3 mL
Tranexamic Acid (15 mg/kg)	NEAT (100 mg/mL)	120 mg	1.2 mL
10% Calcium Chloride (0.2 mL/kg)	NEAT	1.7 mL	1.7 mL

INFUSIONS

Drug	To Make Up in 50 mL	Infusion Rate
Propofol (4 – 12 mg/kg/hr)	NEAT (10 mg/mL)	3 – 10 mL/hr
Morphine (10 – 40 microgram/kg/hr)	8.5 mg (1 mg/kg)	0.5 – 2 mL/hr (1 mL/hr = 20 microgram/kg/hr)
Midazolam (60 – 240 microgram/kg/hr)	50 mg (6 mg/kg)	0.5 – 2 mL/hr (1 mL/hr = 120 microgram/kg/hr)
Noradrenaline / Adrenaline (0.01 – 0.5 microgram/kg/min)	2.5 mg (0.3 mg/kg) in 5% Dextrose	0.1 – 5 mL/hr (1 mL/hr = 0.1 microgram/kg/min)

AGE : 1 year

Wt :	9 – 10 kg	HR :	100 – 150	RR :	25 – 35	Systolic BP :	80 – 95

AIRWAY

OP Airway : Size : 00 – 0	**ET Tube :** Diameter : Cuffed:	3.5
	Uncuffed:	4.5
LMA : Size : 2	Length (Oral) :	12.5 cm

CARDIAC

Defibrillation (4 J/kg)	50 J		**IV – Arrest** (10 microgram/kg)	1.0 mL (1 in 10,000)
Atropine (20 microgram/kg)	200 microgram	**Adrenaline**	**IM – Anaphylaxis** (10 microgram/kg)	1.0 mL (1 in 10,000)
Amiodarone (5 mg/kg)	50 mg (1.7 mL of minijet)		**Nebulised – Croup** (400 microgram/kg)	4.0 mL (1 in 1,000)

FLUIDS

Crystalloids :	Trauma (10 mL/kg): Other (20 mL/kg) :	100 mL 200 mL	Blood, FFP or Platelets (10 mL/kg)	100 mL
10% Dextrose : (Hypoglycaemia) (2 mL/kg)		20 mL	Mannitol 20% (0.25 – 0.5 g/kg)	12 – 25 mL (0.5 g/kg = 2.5 mL/kg)

DRUGS

Drug (Dose)	Neat or Dilution (mg/mL)	Calculated Dose (10 kg)	Volume to be given (mL)
Propofol (1 – 4 mg/kg)	NEAT (10 mg/mL)	10 – 40 mg	1 – 4 mL
Ketamine IV (2 mg/kg)	NEAT (10 mg/mL)	20 mg	2 mL
Fentanyl (1 – 2 microgram/kg)	Dilute to 10 microgram/mL	10 – 20 microgram	1 – 2 mL
Morphine (0.1 mg/kg)	Dilute to 1 mg/mL	1 mg (Repeat PRN)	1 mL
Paracetamol IV (15 mg/kg)	NEAT (10 mg/mL)	150 mg	15 mL
Suxamethonium (2 mg/kg)	Dilute to 10 mg/mL	20 mg	2 mL
Rocuronium (1 mg/kg)	NEAT (10 mg/mL)	10 mg	1 mL
Atracurium (0.5 mg/kg)	NEAT (10 mg/mL)	5 mg	0.5 mL
Sugammadex (16 mg/kg)	NEAT (100 mg/mL)	150 mg	1.5 mL
Tranexamic Acid (15 mg/kg)	NEAT (100 mg/mL)	150 mg	1.5 mL
10% Calcium Chloride (0.2 mL/kg)	NEAT	2 mL	2 mL

INFUSIONS

Drug	To Make Up in 50 mL	Infusion Rate
Propofol (4 – 12 mg/kg/hr)	NEAT (10 mg/mL)	4 – 12 mL/hr
Morphine (10 – 40 microgram/kg/hr)	10 mg (1 mg/kg)	0.5 – 2 mL/hr (1 mL/hr = 20 microgram/kg/hr)
Midazolam (60 – 240 microgram/kg/hr)	60 mg (6 mg/kg)	0.5 – 2 mL/hr (1 mL/hr = 120 microgram/kg/hr)
Noradrenaline / Adrenaline (0.01 – 0.5 microgram/kg/min)	3 mg (0.3 mg/kg) in 5% Dextrose	0.1 – 5 mL/hr (1 mL/hr = 0.1 microgram/kg/min)

AGE : 18 months

Wt :	10 – 11 kg	HR :	100 – 150	RR :	25 – 35	Systolic BP :	80 – 95

AIRWAY

OP Airway : Size : 00 – 0	ET Tube :	
	Diameter : Cuffed:	3.5
	Uncuffed:	4.5
LMA : Size : 2	Length (Oral) :	12.5 – 13 cm

CARDIAC

Defibrillation (4 J/kg)	50 J	Adrenaline	IV – Arrest (10 microgram/kg)	1.1 mL (1 in 10,000)
Atropine (20 microgram/kg)	220 microgram		IM – Anaphylaxis (10 microgram/kg)	0.11 mL (1 in 1,000)
Amiodarone (5 mg/kg)	55 mg (1.8 mL of minijet)		Nebulised – Croup (400 microgram/kg)	4.4 mL (1 in 1,000)

FLUIDS

Crystalloids :	Trauma (10 mL/kg): Other (20 mL/kg) :	110 mL 220 mL	Blood, FFP or Platelets (10 mL/kg)	110 mL
10% Dextrose : (Hypoglycaemia) (2 mL/kg)		22 mL	Mannitol 20% (0.25 – 0.5 g/kg)	14 – 28 mL (0.5 g/kg = 2.5 mL/kg)

DRUGS

Drug (Dose)	Neat or Dilution (mg/mL)	Calculated Dose (11 kg)	Volume to be given (mL)
Propofol (1 – 4 mg/kg)	NEAT (10 mg/mL)	10 – 45 mg	1 – 4.5 mL
Ketamine IV (2 mg/kg)	NEAT (10 mg/mL)	25 mg	2.5 mL
Fentanyl (1 – 2 microgram/kg)	Dilute to 10 microgram/mL	10 – 20 microgram	1 – 2 mL
Morphine (0.1 mg/kg)	Dilute to 1 mg/mL	1 mg (Repeat PRN)	1 mL
Paracetamol IV (15 mg/kg)	NEAT (10 mg/mL)	165 mg	16.5 mL
Suxamethonium (2 mg/kg)	Dilute to 10 mg/mL	22 mg	2.2 mL
Rocuronium (1 mg/kg)	NEAT (10 mg/mL)	10 mg	1 mL
Atracurium (0.5 mg/kg)	NEAT (10 mg/mL)	5 mg	0.5 mL
Sugammadex (16 mg/kg)	NEAT (100 mg/mL)	170 mg	1.7 mL
Tranexamic Acid (15 mg/kg)	NEAT (100 mg/mL)	160 mg	1.6 mL
10% Calcium Chloride (0.2 mL/kg)	NEAT	2.2 mL	2.2 mL

INFUSIONS

Drug	To Make Up in 50 mL	Infusion Rate
Propofol (4 – 12 mg/kg/hr)	NEAT (10 mg/mL)	4 – 12 mL/hr
Morphine (10 – 40 microgram/kg/hr)	11 mg (1 mg/mL)	0.5 – 2 mL/hr (1 mL/hr = 20 microgram/kg/hr)
Midazolam (60 – 240 microgram/kg/hr)	60 mg (6 mg/kg)	0.5 – 2 mL/hr (1 mL/hr = 120 microgram/kg/hr)
Noradrenaline / Adrenaline (0.01 – 0.5 microgram/kg/min)	3 mg (0.3 mg/kg) in 5% Dextrose	0.1 – 5 mL/hr (1 mL/hr = 0.1 microgram/kg/min)

AGE : 2 years

Wt : 11 – 12 kg	HR : 95 – 140	RR : 25 – 30	Systolic BP : 80 – 100

AIRWAY

OP Airway : Size : 0 – 1	ET Tube :		4.0
LMA : Size : 2	Diameter : Cuffed:		5.0
	Uncuffed:		
	Length (Oral) :		13 cm

CARDIAC

Defibrillation (4 J/kg)	50 J		IV – Arrest (10 microgram/kg)	1.2 mL (1 in 10,000)
Atropine (20 microgram/kg)	240 microgram	Adrenaline	IM – Anaphylaxis (10 microgram/kg)	0.12 mL (1 in 1,000)
Amiodarone (5 mg/kg)	60 mg (2.0 mL of minijet)		Nebulised – Croup (400 microgram/kg)	4.8 mL (1 in 1,000)

FLUIDS

Crystalloids :	Trauma (10 mL/kg): Other (20 mL/kg) :	120 mL 240 mL	Blood, FFP or Platelets (10 mL/kg)	120 mL
10% Dextrose : (Hypoglycaemia) (2 mL/kg)		24 mL	Mannitol 20% (0.25 – 0.5 g/kg)	15 – 30 mL (0.5 g/kg = 2.5 mL/kg)

DRUGS

Drug (Dose)	Neat or Dilution (mg/mL)	Calculated Dose (12 kg)	Volume to be given (mL)
Propofol (1 – 4 mg/kg)	NEAT (10 mg/mL)	12 – 50 mg	1.2 – 5 mL
Ketamine IV (2 mg/kg)	NEAT (10 mg/mL)	25 mg	2.5 mL
Fentanyl (1 – 2 microgram/kg)	Dilute to 10 microgram/mL	12 – 25 microgram	1.2 – 2.5 mL
Morphine (0.1 mg/kg)	Dilute to 1 mg/mL	1.2 mg (Repeat PRN)	1.2 mL
Paracetamol IV (15 mg/kg)	NEAT (10 mg/mL)	180 mg	18 mL
Suxamethonium (2 mg/kg)	Dilute to 10 mg/mL	24 mg	2.4 mL
Rocuronium (1 mg/kg)	NEAT (10 mg/mL)	12 mg	1.2 mL
Atracurium (0.5 mg/kg)	NEAT (10 mg/mL)	6 mg	0.6 mL
Sugammadex (16 mg/kg)	NEAT (100 mg/mL)	200 mg	2 mL
Tranexamic Acid (15 mg/kg)	NEAT (100 mg/mL)	180 mg	1.8 mL
10% Calcium Chloride (0.2 mL/kg)	NEAT	2.4 mL	2.4 mL

INFUSIONS

Drug	To Make Up in 50 mL	Infusion Rate
Propofol (4 – 12 mg/kg/hr)	NEAT (10 mg/mL)	4 – 14 mL/hr
Morphine (10 – 40 microgram/kg/hr)	12 mg (1 mg/kg)	0.5 – 2 mL/hr (1 mL/hr = 20 microgram/kg/hr)
Midazolam (60 – 240 microgram/kg/hr)	72 mg (6 mg/kg)	0.5 – 2 mL/hr (1 mL/hr = 120 microgram/kg/hr)
Noradrenaline / Adrenaline (0.01 – 0.5 microgram/kg/min)	3.6 mg (0.3 mg/kg) in 5% Dextrose	0.1 – 5 mL/hr (1 mL/hr = 0.1 microgram/kg/min)

AGE : 3 years

Wt : 11 – 15 kg	HR : 95 – 140	RR : 25 – 30	Systolic BP : 80 – 100

AIRWAY

OP Airway : Size : 1	ET Tube :	
	Diameter : Cuffed:	4.0
LMA : Size : 2	Uncuffed:	5.0
	Length (Oral) :	13cm

CARDIAC

Defibrillation (4 J/kg)	70 J	Adrenaline	IV – Arrest (10 microgram/kg)	1.4 mL (1 in 10,000)
Atropine (20 microgram/kg)	280 microgram		IM – Anaphylaxis (10 microgram/kg)	0.14 mL (1 in 1,000)
Amiodarone (5 mg/kg)	70 mg (2.3 mL of minijet)		Nebulised – Croup (400 microgram/kg)	5.0 mL (1 in 1,000) (max)

FLUIDS

Crystalloids :	Trauma (10 mL/kg): Other (20 mL/kg) :	140 mL 280 mL	Blood, FFP or Platelets (10 mL/kg)	140 mL
10% Dextrose : (Hypoglycaemia) (2 mL/kg)		28 mL	Mannitol 20% (0.25 – 0.5 g/kg)	17.5 – 35 mL (0.5 g/kg = 2.5 mL/kg)

DRUGS

Drug (Dose)	Neat or Dilution (mg/mL)	Calculated Dose (14 kg)	Volume to be given (mL)
Propofol (1 – 4 mg/kg)	NEAT (10 mg/mL)	14 – 55 mg	1.5 – 5.5 mL
Ketamine IV (2 mg/kg)	NEAT (10 mg/mL)	30 mg	3 mL
Fentanyl (1 – 2 microgram/kg)	Dilute to 10 microgram/mL	15 – 30 microgram	1.5 – 3 mL
Morphine (0.1 mg/kg)	Dilute to 1 mg/mL	1.4 mg (Repeat PRN)	1.4 mL
Paracetamol IV (15 mg/kg)	NEAT (10 mg/mL)	210 mg	21 mL
Suxamethonium (2 mg/kg)	Dilute to 10 mg/mL	30 mg	3 mL
Rocuronium (1 mg/kg)	NEAT (10 mg/mL)	15 mg	1.5 mL
Atracurium (0.5 mg/kg)	NEAT (10 mg/mL)	7 mg	0.7 mL
Sugammadex (16 mg/kg)	NEAT (100 mg/mL)	225 mg	2.25 mL
Tranexamic Acid (15 mg/kg)	NEAT (100 mg/mL)	210 mg	2.1 mL
10% Calcium Chloride (0.2 mL/kg)	NEAT	2.8 mL	2.8 mL

INFUSIONS

Drug	To Make Up in 50 mL	Infusion Rate
Propofol (4 – 12 mg/kg/hr)	NEAT (10 mg/mL)	5 – 16 mL/hr
Morphine (10 – 40 microgram/kg/hr)	14 mg (1 mg/kg)	0.5 – 2 mL/hr (1 mL/hr = 20 microgram/kg/hr)
Midazolam (60 – 240 microgram/kg/hr)	84 mg (6 mg/kg)	0.5 – 2 mL/hr (1 mL/hr = 120 microgram/kg/hr)
Noradrenaline / Adrenaline (0.01 – 0.5 microgram/kg/min)	4.2 mg (0.3 mg/kg) in 5% Dextrose	0.1 – 5 mL/hr (1 mL/hr = 0.1 microgram/kg/min)

AGE : 4 years

Wt : 14 – 16 kg	HR : 95 – 150	RR : 25 – 30	Systolic BP : 80 – 100

AIRWAY

OP Airway : Size : 1	ET Tube :		
	Diameter :	Cuffed:	4.5
LMA : Size : 2		Uncuffed:	5.5
	Length (Oral) :		14 cm

CARDIAC

Defibrillation (4 J/kg)	70 J	Adrenaline	IV – Arrest (10 microgram/kg)	1.6 mL (1 in 10,000)
Atropine (20 microgram/kg)	320 microgram		IM – Anaphylaxis (10 microgram/kg)	0.16 mL (1 in 1,000)
Amiodarone (5 mg/kg)	80 mg (2.7 mL of minijet)		Nebulised – Croup (400 microgram/kg)	5.0 mL (1 in 1,000) (max)

FLUIDS

Crystalloids :	Trauma (10 mL/kg): Other (20 mL/kg) :	160 mL 320 mL	Blood, FFP or Platelets (10 mL/kg)	160 mL
10% Dextrose : (Hypoglycaemia) (2 mL/kg)		32 mL	Mannitol 20% (0.25 – 0.5 g/kg)	20 – 40 mL (0.5 g/kg = 2.5 mL/kg)

DRUGS

Drug (Dose)	Neat or Dilution (mg/mL)	Calculated Dose (16 kg)	Volume to be given (mL)
Propofol (1 – 4 mg/kg)	NEAT (10 mg/mL)	15 – 65 mg	1.5 – 6.5 mL
Ketamine IV (2 mg/kg)	NEAT (10 mg/mL)	30 mg	3 mL
Fentanyl (1 – 2 microgram/kg)	Dilute to 10 microgram/mL	15 – 30 microgram	1.5 – 3 mL
Morphine (0.1 mg/kg)	Dilute to 1 mg/mL	1.5 mg (Repeat PRN)	1.5 mL
Paracetamol IV (15 mg/kg)	NEAT (10 mg/mL)	240 mg	24 mL
Suxamethonium (2 mg/kg)	Dilute to 10 mg/mL	30 mg	3 mL
Rocuronium (1 mg/kg)	NEAT (10 mg/mL)	15 mg	1.5 mL
Atracurium (0.5 mg/kg)	NEAT (10 mg/mL)	10 mg	1 mL
Sugammadex (16 mg/kg)	NEAT (100 mg/mL)	250 mg	2.5 mL
Tranexamic Acid (15 mg/kg)	NEAT (100 mg/mL)	240 mg	2.4 mL
10% Calcium Chloride (0.2 mL/kg)	NEAT	3.2 mL	3.2 mL

INFUSIONS

Drug	To Make Up in 50 mL	Infusion Rate
Propofol (4 – 12 mg/kg/hr)	NEAT (10 mg/mL)	6 – 18 mL/hr
Morphine (10 – 40 microgram/kg/hr)	16 mg (1 mg/kg)	0.5 – 2 mL/hr (1 mL/hr = 20 microgram/kg/hr)
Midazolam (60 – 240 microgram/kg/hr)	96 mg (6 mg/kg)	0.5 – 2 mL/hr (1 mL/hr = 120 microgram/kg/hr)
Noradrenaline / Adrenaline (0.01 – 0.5 microgram/kg/min)	4.5 mg (0.3 mg/kg) in 5% Dextrose	0.1 – 5 mL/hr (1 mL/hr = 0.1 microgram/kg/min)

AGE : 5 years

| Wt : 16 – 22 kg | HR : 90 – 130 | RR : 20 – 25 | Systolic BP : 90 – 110 |

AIRWAY

OP Airway : Size : 1	ET Tube :	
	Diameter : Cuffed:	4.5
LMA : Size : 2 – 2.5	Uncuffed:	5.5
	Length (Oral) :	14.5 cm

CARDIAC

Defibrillation (4 J/kg)	70 J	Adrenaline	IV – Arrest (10 microgram/kg)	1.8 mL (1 in 10,000)
Atropine (20 microgram/kg)	360 microgram		IM – Anaphylaxis (10 microgram/kg)	0.18 mL (1 in 1,000)
Amiodarone (5 mg/kg)	90 mg (3 mL of minijet)		Nebulised – Croup (400 microgram/kg)	5.0 mL (1 in 1,000) (max)

FLUIDS

Crystalloids :	Trauma (10 mL/kg): Other (20 mL/kg) :	180 mL 360 mL	Blood, FFP or Platelets (10 mL/kg)	180 mL
10% Dextrose : (Hypoglycaemia) (2 mL/kg)		36 mL	Mannitol 20% (0.25 – 0.5 g/kg)	22.5 – 45 mL (0.5 g/kg = 2.5 mL/kg)

DRUGS

Drug (Dose)	Neat or Dilution (mg/mL)	Calculated Dose (18 kg)	Volume to be given (mL)
Propofol (1 – 4 mg/kg)	NEAT (10 mg/mL)	18 – 72 mg	2 – 7 mL
Ketamine IV (2 mg/kg)	NEAT (10 mg/mL)	35 mg	3.5 mL
Fentanyl (1 – 2 microgram/kg)	Dilute to 10 microgram/mL	20 – 40 microgram	2 – 4 mL
Morphine (0.1 mg/kg)	Dilute to 1 mg/mL	1.8 mg (Repeat PRN)	1.8 mL
Paracetamol IV (15 mg/kg)	NEAT (10 mg/mL)	270 mg	27 mL
Suxamethonium (2 mg/kg)	Dilute to 10 mg/mL	35 mg	3.5 mL
Rocuronium (1 mg/kg)	NEAT (10 mg/mL)	20 mg	2 mL
Atracurium (0.5 mg/kg)	NEAT (10 mg/mL)	10 mg	1 mL
Sugammadex (16 mg/kg)	NEAT (100 mg/mL)	290 mg	2.9 mL
Tranexamic Acid (15 mg/kg)	NEAT (100 mg/mL)	270 mg	2.7 mL
10% Calcium Chloride (0.2 mL/kg)	NEAT	3.6 mL	3.6 mL

INFUSIONS

Drug	To Make Up in 50 mL	Infusion Rate
Propofol (4 – 12 mg/kg/hr)	NEAT (10 mg/mL)	7 – 21 mL/hr
Morphine (10 – 40 microgram/kg/hr)	18 mg (1 mg/kg)	0.5 – 2 mL/hr (1 mL/hr = 20 microgram/kg/hr)
Midazolam (60 – 240 microgram/kg/hr)	108 mg (6 mg/kg)	0.5 – 2 mL/hr (1 mL/hr = 120 microgram/kg/hr)
Noradrenaline / Adrenaline (0.01 – 0.5 microgram/kg/min)	5.4 mg (0.3 mg/kg) in 5% Dextrose	0.1 – 5 mL/hr (1 mL/hr = 0.1 microgram/kg/min)

AGE : 6 years

Wt : 20 – 25 kg	HR : 80 – 120	RR : 20 – 25	Systolic BP : 90 – 110

AIRWAY

OP Airway :	Size : 1	ET Tube : Diameter :	Cuffed:	5.0
			Uncuffed:	6.0
LMA :	Size : 2.5	Length (Oral) :		15 cm

CARDIAC

Defibrillation (4 J/kg)	100 J	Adrenaline	IV – Arrest (10 microgram/kg)	2.5 mL (1 in 10,000)
Atropine (20 microgram/kg)	500 microgram		IM – Anaphylaxis (10 microgram/kg)	0.25 mL (1 in 1,000)
Amiodarone (5 mg/kg)	125 mg (4.2 mL of minijet)		Nebulised – Croup (400 microgram/kg)	5.0 mL (1 in 1,000) (max)

FLUIDS

Crystalloids :	Trauma (10 mL/kg): Other (20 mL/kg) :	250 mL 500 mL	Blood, FFP or Platelets (10 mL/kg)	250 mL
10% Dextrose : (Hypoglycaemia) (2 mL/kg)		50 mL	Mannitol 20% (0.25 – 0.5 g/kg)	30 – 63 mL (0.5 g/kg = 2.5 mL/kg)

DRUGS

Drug (Dose)	Neat or Dilution (mg/mL)	Calculated Dose (25 kg)	Volume to be given (mL)
Propofol (1 – 4 mg/kg)	NEAT (10 mg/mL)	25 – 100 mg	2.5 – 10 mL
Ketamine IV (2 mg/kg)	NEAT (10 mg/mL)	50 mg	5 mL
Fentanyl (1 – 2 microgram/kg)	Dilute to 10 microgram/mL	20 – 50 microgram	2.5 – 5 mL
Morphine (0.1 mg/kg)	Dilute to 1 mg/mL	2.5 mg (Repeat PRN)	2.5 mL
Paracetamol IV (15 mg/kg)	NEAT (10 mg/mL)	380 mg	38 mL
Suxamethonium (2 mg/kg)	Dilute to 10 mg/mL	50 mg	5 mL
Rocuronium (1 mg/kg)	NEAT (10 mg/mL)	25 mg	2.5 mL
Atracurium (0.5 mg/kg)	NEAT (10 mg/mL)	13 mg	1.3 mL
Sugammadex (16 mg/kg)	NEAT (100 mg/mL)	400 mg	4 mL
Tranexamic Acid (15 mg/kg)	NEAT (100 mg/mL)	380 mg	3.8 mL
10% Calcium Chloride (0.2 mL/kg)	NEAT	5 mL	5 mL

INFUSIONS

Drug	To Make Up in 50 mL	Infusion Rate
Propofol (4 – 12 mg/kg/hr)	NEAT (10 mg/mL)	10 – 30 mL/hr
Morphine (10 – 40 microgram/kg/hr)	25 mg (1 mg/kg)	0.5 – 2 mL/hr (1 mL/hr = 20 microgram/kg/hr)
Midazolam (60 – 240 microgram/kg/hr)	150 mg (6 mg/kg)	0.5 – 2 mL/hr (1 mL/hr = 120 microgram/kg/hr)
Noradrenaline / Adrenaline (0.01 – 0.5 microgram/kg/min)	7.5 mg (0.3 mg/kg) in 5% Dextrose	0.1 – 5 mL/hr (1 mL/hr = 0.1 microgram/kg/min)

AGE : 7 years

Wt : 22 – 30 kg	HR : 80 – 120	RR : 20 – 25	Systolic BP : 90 – 110

AIRWAY

OP Airway : Size : 1 – 2	ET Tube :	
	Diameter : Cuffed:	5.0
LMA : Size : 2.5	Uncuffed:	6.0
	Length (Oral) :	15 cm

CARDIAC

Defibrillation (4 J/kg)	125 J		IV – Arrest (10 microgram/kg)	2.8 mL (1 in 10,000)
Atropine (20 microgram/kg)	560 microgram	Adrenaline	IM – Anaphylaxis (10 microgram/kg)	0.28 mL (1 in 1,000)
Amiodarone (5 mg/kg)	140 mg (4.6 mL of minijet)		Nebulised – Croup (400 microgram/kg)	5.0 mL (1 in 1,000) (max)

FLUIDS

Crystalloids :	Trauma (10 mL/kg): Other (20 mL/kg) :	280 mL 560 mL	Blood, FFP or Platelets (10 mL/kg)	280 mL
10% Dextrose : (Hypoglycaemia) (2 mL/kg)		56 mL	Mannitol 20% (0.25 – 0.5 g/kg)	35 – 70 mL (0.5 g/kg = 2.5 mL/kg)

DRUGS

Drug (Dose)	Neat or Dilution (mg/mL)	Calculated Dose (28 kg)	Volume to be given (mL)
Propofol (1 – 4 mg/kg)	NEAT (10 mg/mL)	30 – 115mg	3 – 11.5 mL
Ketamine IV (2 mg/kg)	NEAT (10 mg/mL)	55 mg	5.5 mL
Fentanyl (1 – 2 microgram/kg)	Dilute to 10 microgram/mL	30 – 55 microgram	3 – 5.5 mL
Morphine (0.1 mg/kg)	Dilute to 1 mg/mL	2.8 mg (Repeat PRN)	2.8 mL
Paracetamol IV (15 mg/kg)	NEAT (10 mg/mL)	420 mg	42 mL
Suxamethonium (2 mg/kg)	Dilute to 10 mg/mL	55 mg	5.5 mL
Rocuronium (1 mg/kg)	NEAT (10 mg/mL)	28 mg	3 mL
Atracurium (0.5 mg/kg)	NEAT (10 mg/mL)	14 mg	1.4 mL
Sugammadex (16 mg/kg)	NEAT (100 mg/mL)	450 mg	4.5 mL
Tranexamic Acid (15 mg/kg)	NEAT (100 mg/mL)	420 mg	4.2 mL
10% Calcium Chloride (0.2 mL/kg)	NEAT	5.6 mL	5.6 mL

INFUSIONS

Drug	To Make Up in 50 mL	Infusion Rate
Propofol (4 – 12 mg/kg/hr)	NEAT (10 mg/mL)	11 – 33 mL/hr
Morphine (10 – 40 microgram/kg/hr)	28 mg (1 mg/kg)	0.5 – 2 mL/hr (1 mL/hr = 20 microgram/kg/hr)
Midazolam (60 – 240 microgram/kg/hr)	168 mg (6 mg/kg)	0.5 – 2 mL/hr (1 mL/hr = 120 microgram/kg/hr)
Noradrenaline / Adrenaline (0.01 – 0.5 microgram/kg/min)	8.4 mg (0.3 mg/kg) in 5% Dextrose	0.1 – 5 mL/hr (1 mL/hr = 0.1 microgram/kg/min)

AGE : 8 years

Wt : 25 – 31 kg	HR : 80 – 120	RR : 20 – 25	Systolic BP : 90 – 110

AIRWAY

OP Airway : Size : 1 – 2	ET Tube :		
	Diameter : Cuffed:		5.5
LMA : Size : 3	Uncuffed:		6.5
	Length (Oral) :		16 cm

CARDIAC

Defibrillation (4 J/kg)	125 J		IV – Arrest (10 microgram/kg)	3.0 mL (1 in 10,000)
Atropine (20 microgram/kg)	600 microgram (max)	Adrenaline	IM – Anaphylaxis (10 microgram/kg)	0.3 mL (1 in 1,000)
Amiodarone (5 mg/kg)	150 mg (5.0 mL of minijet)		Nebulised – Croup (400 microgram/kg)	5.0 mL (1 in 1,000) (max)

FLUIDS

Crystalloids :	Trauma (10 mL/kg): Other (20 mL/kg) :	300 mL 600 mL	Blood, FFP or Platelets (10 mL/kg)	300 mL
10% Dextrose : (Hypoglycaemia) (2 mL/kg)		60 mL	Mannitol 20% (0.25 – 0.5 g/kg)	38 – 75 mL (0.5 g/kg = 2.5 mL/kg)

DRUGS

Drug (Dose)	Neat or Dilution (mg/mL)	Calculated Dose (30 kg)	Volume to be given (mL)
Propofol (1 – 4 mg/kg)	NEAT (10 mg/mL)	30 – 120 mg	3 – 12 mL
Ketamine IV (2 mg/kg)	NEAT (10 mg/mL)	60 mg	6 mL
Fentanyl (1 – 2 microgram/kg)	Dilute to 10 microgram/mL	30 – 60 microgram	3 – 6 mL
Morphine (0.1 mg/kg)	Dilute to 1 mg/mL	3 mg (Repeat PRN)	3 mL
Paracetamol IV (15 mg/kg)	NEAT (10 mg/mL)	450 mg	45 mL
Suxamethonium (2 mg/kg)	Dilute to 10 mg/mL	60 mg	6 mL
Rocuronium (1 mg/kg)	NEAT (10 mg/mL)	30 mg	3 mL
Atracurium (0.5 mg/kg)	NEAT (10 mg/mL)	15 mg	1.5 mL
Sugammadex (16 mg/kg)	NEAT (100 mg/mL)	500 mg	5 mL
Tranexamic Acid (15 mg/kg)	NEAT (100 mg/mL)	450 mg	4.5 mL
10% Calcium Chloride (0.2 mL/kg)	NEAT	6 mL	6 mL

INFUSIONS

Drug	To Make Up in 50 mL	Infusion Rate	
Propofol (4 – 12 mg/kg/hr)	NEAT (10 mg/mL)	12 – 36 mL/hr	
Morphine (10 – 40 microgram/kg/hr)	30 mg (1 mg/kg)	0.5 – 2 mL/hr	(1 mL/hr = 20 microgram/kg/hr)
Midazolam (60 – 240 microgram/kg/hr)	180 mg (6 mg/kg)	0.5 – 2 mL/hr	(1 mL/hr = 120 microgram/kg/hr)
Noradrenaline / Adrenaline (0.01 – 0.5 microgram/kg/min)	9 mg (0.3 mg/kg) in 5% Dextrose	0.1 – 5 mL/hr	(1 mL/hr = 0.1 microgram/kg/min)

AGE : 9 years

Wt : 28 – 35 kg	HR : 80 – 120	RR : 20 – 25	Systolic BP : 90 – 110

AIRWAY

OP Airway : Size : 1 – 2	ET Tube : Diameter : Cuffed:	5.5
LMA : Size : 2.5 – 3	Uncuffed: Length (Oral) :	6.5 / 16.5 cm

CARDIAC

Defibrillation (4 J/kg)	150 J	Adrenaline	IV – Arrest (10 microgram/kg)	3.4 mL (1 in 10,000)
Atropine (20 microgram/kg)	600 microgram (max)		IM – Anaphylaxis (10 microgram/kg)	0.34 mL (1 in 1,000)
Amiodarone (5 mg/kg)	170 mg (5.6 mL of minijet)		Nebulised – Croup (400 microgram/kg)	5.0 mL (1 in 1,000) (max)

FLUIDS

Crystalloids :	Trauma (10 mL/kg): Other (20 mL/kg) :	340 mL 680 mL	Blood, FFP or Platelets (10 mL/kg)	340 mL
10% Dextrose : (Hypoglycaemia) (2 mL/kg)		68 mL	Mannitol 20% (0.25 – 0.5 g/kg)	42 – 85 mL (0.5 g/kg = 2.5 mL/kg)

DRUGS

Drug (Dose)	Neat or Dilution (mg/mL)	Calculated Dose (34 kg)	Volume to be given (mL)
Propofol (1 – 4 mg/kg)	NEAT (10 mg/mL)	35 – 140 mg	3.5 – 14 mL
Ketamine IV (2 mg/kg)	NEAT (10 mg/mL)	70 mg	7 mL
Fentanyl (1 – 2 microgram/kg)	Dilute to 10 microgram/mL	35 – 70 microgram	3.5 – 7 mL
Morphine (0.1 mg/kg)	Dilute to 1 mg/mL	3.4 mg (Repeat PRN)	3.4 mL
Paracetamol IV (15 mg/kg)	NEAT (10 mg/mL)	500 mg	50 mL
Suxamethonium (2 mg/kg)	Dilute to 10 mg/mL	70 mg	7 mL
Rocuronium (1 mg/kg)	NEAT (10 mg/mL)	35 mg	3.5 mL
Atracurium (0.5 mg/kg)	NEAT (10 mg/mL)	17 mg	1.7 mL
Sugammadex (16 mg/kg)	NEAT (100 mg/mL)	550 mg	5.5 mL
Tranexamic Acid (15 mg/kg)	NEAT (100 mg/mL)	500 mg	50 mL
10% Calcium Chloride (0.2 mL/kg)	NEAT	6.8 mL	6.8 mL

INFUSIONS

Drug	To Make Up in 50 mL	Infusion Rate
Propofol (4 – 12 mg/kg/hr)	NEAT (10 mg/mL)	13 – 40 mL/hr
Morphine (10 – 40 microgram/kg/hr)	34 mg (1 mg/mL)	0.5 – 2 mL/hr (1 mL/hr = 20 microgram/kg/hr)
Midazolam (60 – 240 microgram/kg/hr)	204 mg (6 mg/mL)	0.5 – 2 mL/hr (1 mL/hr = 120 microgram/kg/hr)
Noradrenaline / Adrenaline (0.01 – 0.5 microgram/kg/min)	10.2 mg (0.3 mg/mL) in 5% Dextrose	0.1 – 5 mL/hr (1 mL/hr = 0.1 microgram/kg/min)

AGE : 10 years

Wt : 30 – 37 kg	HR : 80 – 120	RR : 20 – 25	Systolic BP : 90 – 110

AIRWAY

OP Airway :	Size : 2 – 3	ET Tube :		
		Diameter :	Cuffed:	6.0
			Uncuffed:	7.0
LMA :	Size : 3	Length (Oral) :		17 cm

CARDIAC

Defibrillation (4 J/kg)	150 J	Adrenaline	IV – Arrest (10 microgram/kg)	3.7 mL (1 in 10,000)
Atropine (20 microgram/kg)	600 microgram (max)		IM – Anaphylaxis (10 microgram/kg)	0.37 mL (1 in 1,000)
Amiodarone (5 mg/kg)	185 mg (6.1 mL of minijet)		Nebulised – Croup (400 microgram/kg)	5.0 mL (1 in 1,000) (max)

FLUIDS

Crystalloids :	Trauma (10 mL/kg): Other (20 mL/kg) :	370 mL 740 mL	Blood, FFP or Platelets (10 mL/kg)	370 mL
10% Dextrose : (Hypoglycaemia) (2 mL/kg)		74 mL	Mannitol 20% (0.25 – 0.5 g/kg)	46 – 92 mL (0.5 g/kg = 2.5 mL/kg)

DRUGS

Drug (Dose)	Neat or Dilution (mg/mL)	Calculated Dose (37 kg)	Volume to be given (mL)
Propofol (1 – 4 mg/kg)	NEAT (10 mg/mL)	37 – 150 mg	3.7 – 15 mL
Ketamine IV (2 mg/kg)	NEAT (10 mg/mL)	75 mg	7.5 mL
Fentanyl (1 – 2 microgram/kg)	Dilute to 10 microgram/mL	37 – 75 microgram	3.7 – 7.5 mL
Morphine (0.1 mg/kg)	Dilute to 1 mg/mL	3.7 mg (Repeat PRN)	3.7 mL
Paracetamol IV (15 mg/kg)	NEAT (10 mg/mL)	555 mg	55.5 mL
Suxamethonium (2 mg/kg)	Dilute to 10 mg/mL	75 mg	7.5 mL
Rocuronium (1 mg/kg)	NEAT (10 mg/mL)	37 mg	3.7 mL
Atracurium (0.5 mg/kg)	NEAT (10 mg/mL)	18 mg	1.8 mL
Sugammadex (16 mg/kg)	NEAT (100 mg/mL)	590 mg	5.9 mL
Tranexamic Acid (15 mg/kg)	NEAT (100 mg/mL)	555 mg	5.6 mL
10% Calcium Chloride (0.2 mL/kg)	NEAT	7.5 mL	7.5 mL

INFUSIONS

Drug	To Make Up in 50 mL	Infusion Rate
Propofol (4 – 12 mg/kg/hr)	NEAT (10 mg/mL)	14 – 42 mL/hr
Morphine (10 – 40 microgram/kg/hr)	37 mg (1 mg/kg)	0.5 – 2 mL/hr (1 mL/hr = 20 microgram/kg/hr)
Midazolam (60 – 240 microgram/kg/hr)	222 mg (6 mg/kg)	0.5 – 2 mL/hr (1 mL/hr = 120 microgram/kg/hr)
Noradrenaline / Adrenaline (0.01 – 0.5 microgram/kg/min)	11.1 mg (0.3 mg/kg) in 5% Dextrose	0.1 – 5 mL/hr (1 mL/hr = 0.1 microgram/kg/min)

AGE : 11 years

Wt : 31 – 45 kg	HR : 60 – 100	RR : 15 – 20	Systolic BP : 100 – 120

AIRWAY

OP Airway :	Size : 3 – 4	ET Tube : Diameter :	Cuffed:	6.0
			Uncuffed:	7.0
LMA :	Size : 3	Length (Oral) :		17 cm

CARDIAC

Defibrillation (4 J/kg)	175 J		IV – Arrest (10 microgram/kg)	4.0 mL (1 in 10,000)
Atropine (20 microgram/kg)	600 microgram (max)	Adrenaline	IM – Anaphylaxis (10 microgram/kg)	0.4 mL (1 in 1,000)
Amiodarone (5 mg/kg)	200 mg (6.7 mL of minijet)		Nebulised – Croup (400 microgram/kg)	5.0 mL (1 in 1,000) (max)

FLUIDS

Crystalloids :	Trauma (10 mL/kg): Other (20 mL/kg) :	400 mL 800 mL	Blood, FFP or Platelets (10 mL/kg)	400 mL
10% Dextrose : (Hypoglycaemia) (2 mL/kg)		80 mL	Mannitol 20% (0.25 – 0.5 g/kg)	50 – 100 mL (0.5 g/kg = 2.5 mL/kg)

DRUGS

Drug (Dose)	Neat or Dilution (mg/mL)	Calculated Dose (40 kg)	Volume to be given (mL)
Propofol (1 – 4 mg/kg)	NEAT (10 mg/mL)	40 – 160 mg	4 – 16 mL
Ketamine IV (2 mg/kg)	NEAT (10 mg/mL)	80 mg	8 mL
Fentanyl (1 – 2 microgram/kg)	Dilute to 10 microgram/mL	40 – 80 microgram	4 – 8 mL
Morphine (0.1 mg/kg)	Dilute to 1 mg/mL	4 mg (Repeat PRN)	4 mL
Paracetamol IV (15 mg/kg)	NEAT (10 mg/mL)	600 mg	60 mL
Suxamethonium (2 mg/kg)	Dilute to 10 mg/mL	80 mg	8 mL
Rocuronium (1 mg/kg)	NEAT (10 mg/mL)	40 mg	4 mL
Atracurium (0.5 mg/kg)	NEAT (10 mg/mL)	20 mg	2 mL
Sugammadex (16 mg/kg)	NEAT (100 mg/mL)	650 mg	6.5 mL
Tranexamic Acid (15 mg/kg)	NEAT (100 mg/mL)	600 mg	6 mL
10% Calcium Chloride (0.2 mL/kg)	NEAT	8 mL	8 mL

INFUSIONS

Drug	To Make Up in 50 mL	Infusion Rate
Propofol (4 – 12 mg/kg/hr)	NEAT (10 mg/mL)	16 – 48 mL/hr
Morphine (10 – 40 microgram/kg/hr)	40 mg (1 mg/kg)	0.5 – 2 mL/hr (1 mL/hr = 20 microgram/kg/hr)
Midazolam (60 – 240 microgram/kg/hr)	240 mg (6 mg/kg)	0.5 – 2 mL/hr (1 mL/hr = 120 microgram/kg/hr)
Noradrenaline / Adrenaline (0.01 – 0.5 microgram/kg/min)	12 mg (0.3 mg/kg) in 5% Dextrose	0.1 – 5 mL/hr (1 mL/hr = 0.1 microgram/kg/min)

AGE : 12 years

Wt :	32 – 50 kg	HR :	60 – 100	RR :	15 – 20	Systolic BP :	100 – 120

AIRWAY

OP Airway :	Size : 3 – 4	ET Tube :		
		Diameter :	Cuffed:	6.5
			Uncuffed:	7.5
LMA :	Size : 3	Length (Oral) :		18 cm

CARDIAC

Defibrillation (4 J/kg)	175 J		IV – Arrest (10 microgram/kg)	4.3 mL (1 in 10,000)
Atropine (20 microgram/kg)	600 microgram (max)	Adrenaline	IM – Anaphylaxis (10 microgram/kg)	0.43 mL (1 in 1,000)
Amiodarone (5 mg/kg)	215 mg (7.1 mL of minijet)		Nebulised – Croup (400 microgram/kg)	5.0 mL (1 in 1,000) (max)

FLUIDS

Crystalloids :	Trauma (10 mL/kg): Other (20 mL/kg) :	430 mL 860 mL	Blood, FFP or Platelets (10 mL/kg)	430 mL
10% Dextrose : (Hypoglycaemia) (2 mL/kg)		86 mL	Mannitol 20% (0.25 – 0.5 g/kg)	53 – 107 mL (0.5 g/kg = 2.5 mL/kg)

DRUGS

Drug (Dose)	Neat or Dilution (mg/mL)	Calculated Dose (43 kg)	Volume to be given (mL)
Propofol (1 – 4 mg/kg)	NEAT (10 mg/mL)	40 – 170 mg	4 – 17 mL
Ketamine IV (2 mg/kg)	NEAT (10 mg/mL)	85 mg	8.5 mL
Fentanyl (1 – 2 microgram/kg)	Dilute to 10 microgram/mL	40 – 80 microgram	4 – 8 mL
Morphine (0.1 mg/kg)	Dilute to 1 mg/mL	4.3 mg (Repeat PRN)	4.3 mL
Paracetamol IV (15 mg/kg)	NEAT (10 mg/mL)	650 mg	65 mL
Suxamethonium (2 mg/kg)	Dilute to 10 mg/mL	85 mg	8.5 mL
Rocuronium (1 mg/kg)	NEAT (10 mg/mL)	45 mg	4.5 mL
Atracurium (0.5 mg/kg)	NEAT (10 mg/mL)	21 mg	2.1 mL
Sugammadex (16 mg/kg)	NEAT (100 mg/mL)	690 mg	6.9 mL
Tranexamic Acid (15 mg/kg)	NEAT (100 mg/mL)	650 mg	6.5 mL
10% Calcium Chloride (0.2 mL/kg)	NEAT	8.6 mL	8.6 mL

INFUSIONS

Drug	To Make Up in 50 mL	Infusion Rate
Propofol (4 – 12 mg/kg/hr)	NEAT (10 mg/mL)	17 – 51 mL/hr
Morphine (10 – 40 microgram/kg/hr)	43 mg (1 mg/kg)	0.5 – 2 mL/hr (1 mL/hr = 20 microgram/kg/hr)
Midazolam (60 – 240 microgram/kg/hr)	258 mg (6 mg/kg)	0.5 – 2 mL/hr (1 mL/hr = 120 microgram/kg/hr)
Noradrenaline / Adrenaline (0.01 – 0.5 microgram/kg/min)	12.9 mg (0.3 mg/kg) in 5% Dextrose	0.1 – 5 mL/hr (1 mL/hr = 0.1 microgram/kg/min)

PAEDIATRIC CARDIAC ARREST ALGORITHM

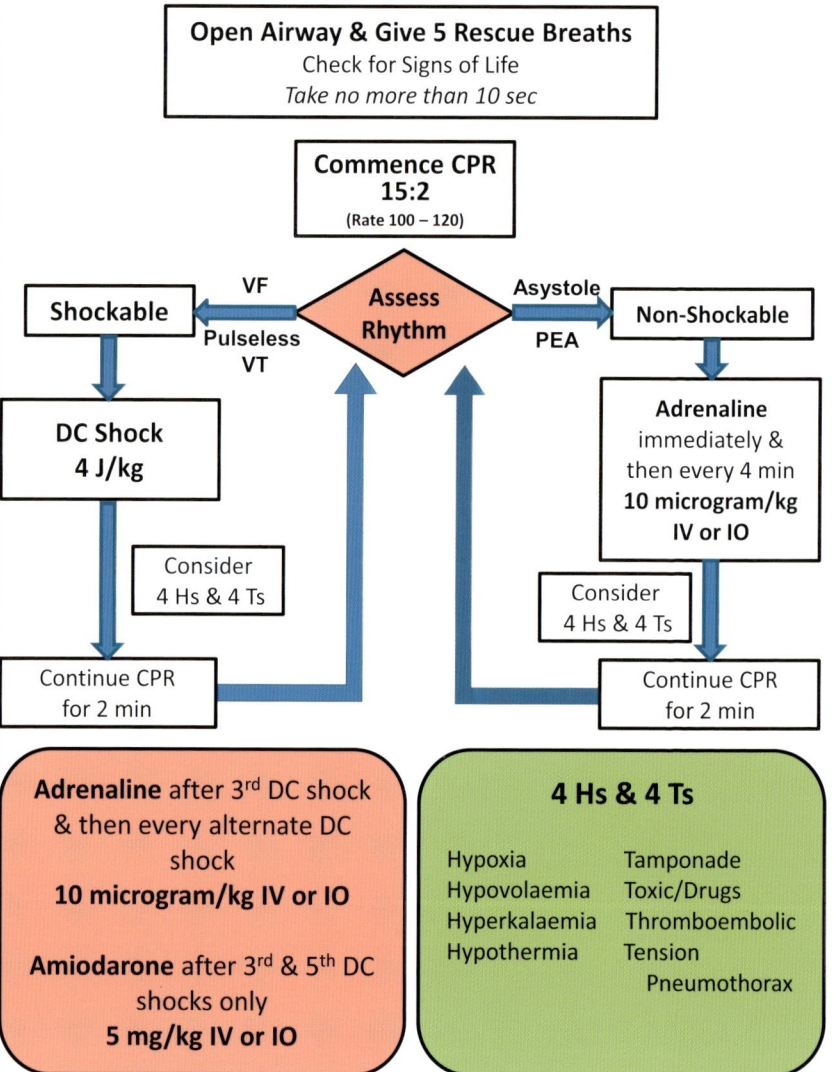

NEWBORN CARDIAC ARREST ALGORITHM

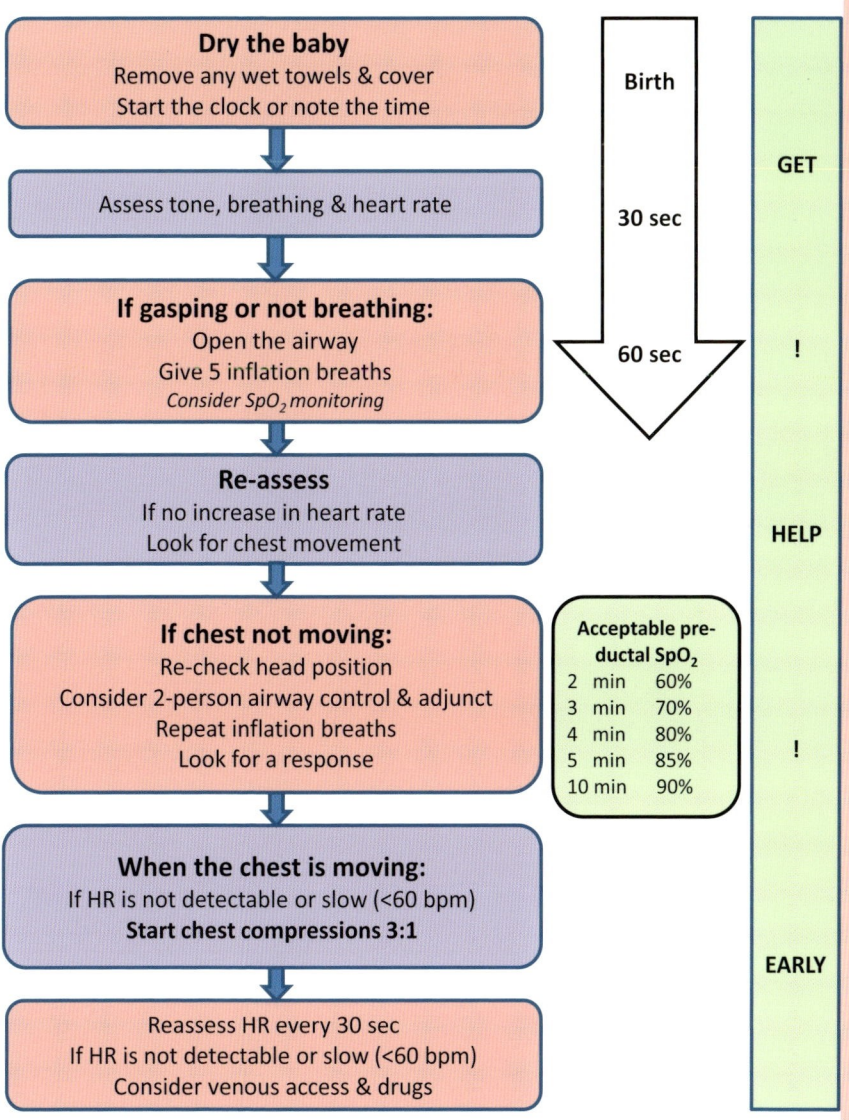

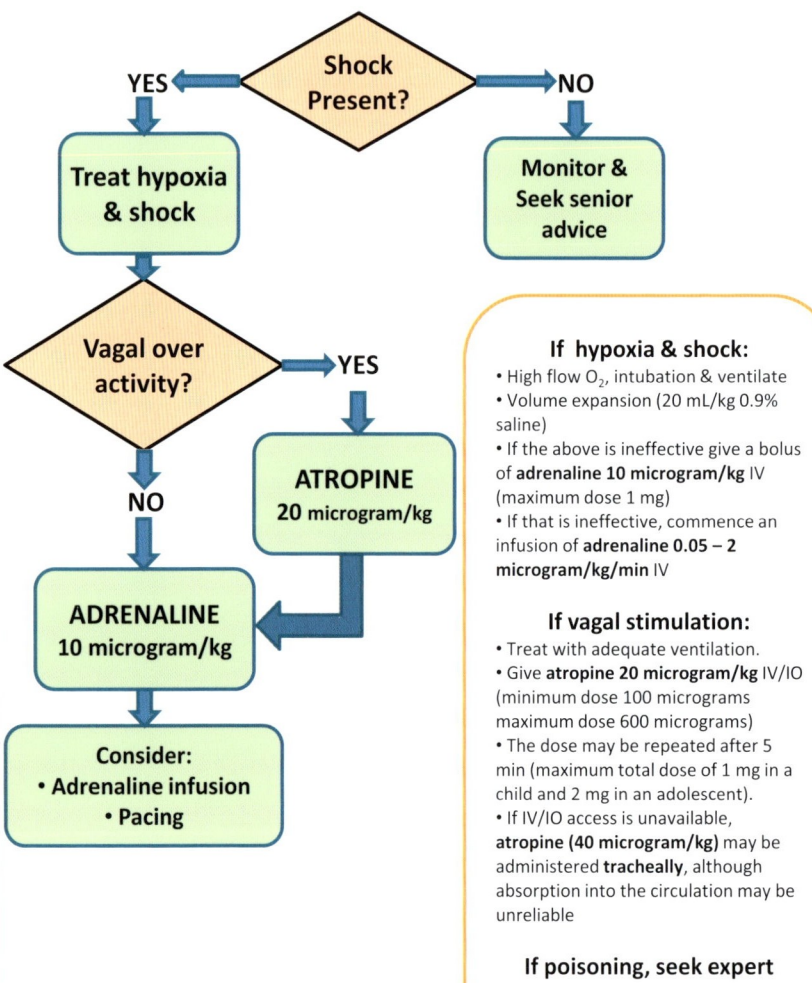

MANAGEMENT OF SVT

SVT in infants generally produces an HR > 220 bpm, and often 250 – 300 bpm

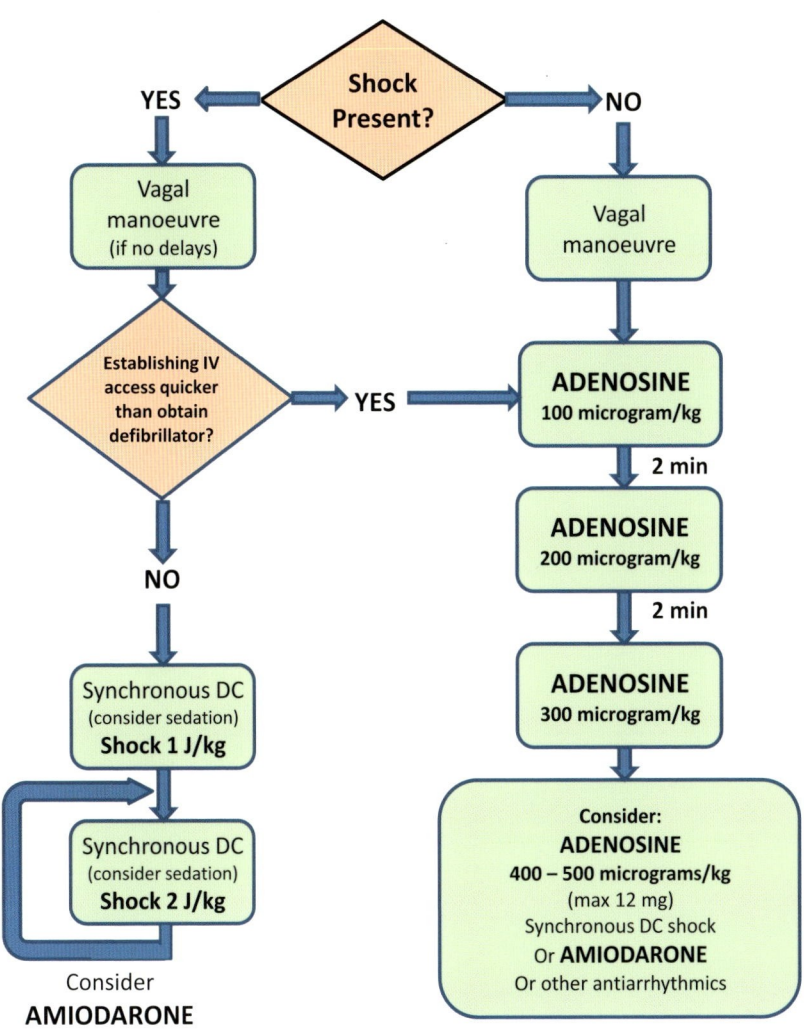

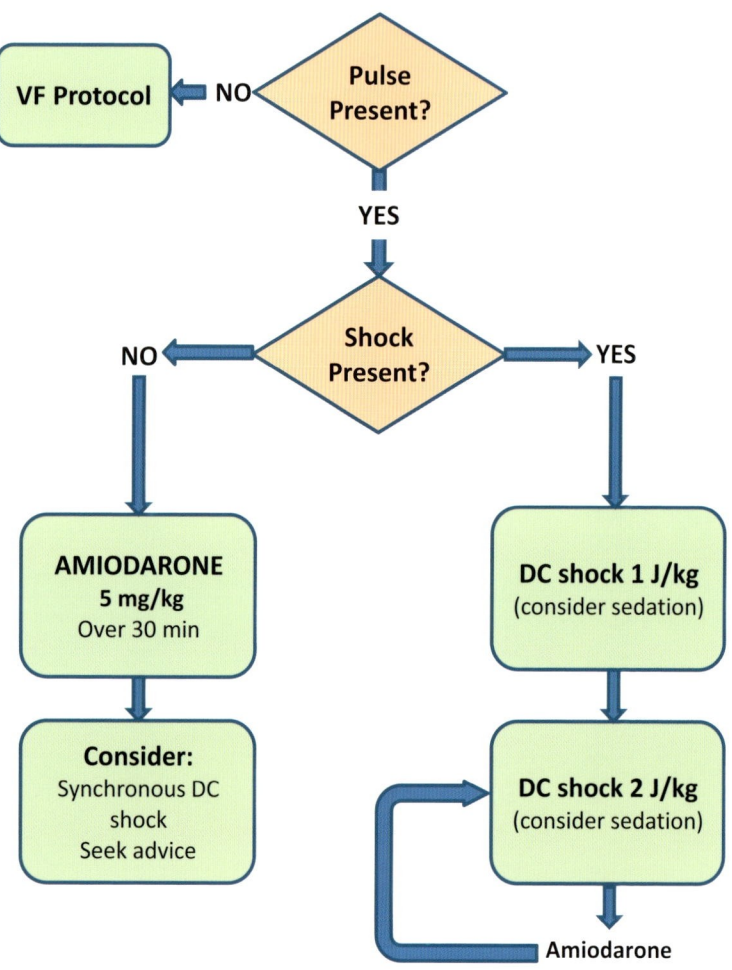

PERI-ARREST DRUGS (1)

INDICATION	ROUTE	AGE/WEIGHT		CAUTION
ADENOSINE Anti-arrhythmic to terminate SVT & to elucidate mechanism of tachycardia	IV bolus	Birth – 12 yrs 100 microgram/kg Increase after 2 min to 200 microgram/kg then 300 microgram/kg	12 – 18 yrs 3 mg 6 mg 12 mg	Heart block Sick sinus Asthma Prolonged QT
ADRENALINE CPR Low CO	IV bolus IV infusion	1 month – 12 yrs 10 microgram/kg 0.01 – 1 microgram/kg/min	12 – 18 yrs 1 mg	
AMIODARONE Arrhythmias	IV loading dose IV infusion	Birth – 18 years 5 mg/kg over 20 – 30 min (max dose 300 mg) (if CPR give over 3 min) 300 microgram/kg/hr (max 1.5 mg/kg/hr as needed) In 5% glucose only		 Do not exceed 1.2 g in 24 hours
ATROPINE Pre-intubation dose or bradycardia induced by vagal stimulation	IV bolus	Birth – 1 mth 1 mth – 12 yrs 12 – 18 yrs 15 microgram/kg 20 microgram/kg 300 microgram – 1 mg (min 100 microgram max 600 microgram)		
CALCIUM GLUCONATE CPR when there is electrolyte disturbance or septicaemia where there is hypocalcaemia	IV bolus	Birth – 18 yrs 0.3 mL/kg of 10% solution Max dose 20 mL (4.5 mmol)		Tissue damage if extravasates
FLECAINIDE Treatment of resistant re-entry SVT, VEs or VT	IV bolus	Birth – 18 yrs 2 mg/kg over 10 min Max dose 150 mg		Avoid in pre-existing Heart Block

PERI-ARREST DRUGS (2)

INDICATION	ROUTE	AGE/WEIGHT		CAUTION
FLUMAZENIL Reversal of acute benzodiazepine overdose	IV bolus	Birth – 12 yrs 10 microgram/kg max 200 microgram (repeat as needed, up to 5 times)	12 – 18 yrs 200 microgram	Limited experience of use in children
LIDOCAINE Antiarrhythmic VF or pulseless VT	IV bolus	Birth – 12 yrs 1 mg/kg max 100 mg Repeat every 5 min to a maximum dose of 3 mg/kg	12 – 18 yrs 50 – 100 mg	
MAGNESIUM SULPHATE Treatment of Torsades de pointes	IV bolus	Birth – 1 month Not Recommended	1 month – 18 yrs 0.1 – 0.2 mmol/kg max 8 mmol	
NALOXONE Reversal of opioid induced central & respiratory depression	IV bolus IV infusion	Birth – 1 mth - 10 microgram/kg	1 mth – 12 yrs 10 microgram/kg Then: 100 microgram/kg 5 – 20 microgram/kg/hr	12 – 18 yrs 10 microgram/kg Then: 2 mg Short half-life
SODIUM BICARBONATE Prolonged cardiac arrest Metabolic acidosis Renal hyperkalaemia	Slow IV	Birth – 18 yrs 1 mL/kg of 8.4% Followed by 0.5 mL/kg of 8.4% if needed 1 – 2 mmol/kg 1 mmol/kg		

TREATMENT OF HYPERKALAEMIA ($K^+ > 6.5$)

If arrhythmia: **0.5 mL/kg 10% Calcium Gluconate** (max 20 mL)
Normal ECG: **2.5 – 10 mg Nebulised Salbutamol** & Repeat serum K^+
    If K^+ falling:
    - **1 g/kg Calcium Resonium** PO/PR & plan dialysis if necessary
    If K^+ remains high:
    - Assess pH: <7.34   **1 – 2 mL/kg 8.4% Sodium Bicarbonate** & Repeat serum K^+
                    >7.35   **5 mL/kg/hr 10% Glucose** & **0.05 units/kg/hr Insulin**
                          (5 units/kg Insulin in 50 mL 0.9% saline. 1 mL/hr = 0.1 units/kg/hr)

MANAGEMENT OF MASSIVE HAEMORRHAGE

Definition of Massive Haemorrhage
- Ongoing severe bleeding & received 20 mL/kg Red Cells or 40 mL/kg of any fluid in preceding hour
- Signs of hypovolaemia +/- coagulopathy

Activate Massive Haemorrhage Protocol
Contact Haematologist (may be initiated by Blood Bank)

→ Resuscitate
→ Haemorrhage control

Take blood & send samples to lab (by hand)
X Match, FBC, Coagulation, Fibrinogen, U+E, Ca^{2+}

Dosing Guide
Red cells	10 – 20 mL/kg
FFP/Octaplas	10 – 20 mL/kg
Platelets	10 – 20 mL/kg
Cryoprecipitate	5 – 10 mL/kg
10% Calcium Chloride	0.2 mL/kg

Tranexamic Acid
(15 mg/kg IV bolus (max 1 g) then 2 mg/kg/hr infusion)

Collect & Transfuse Red Cells (20 mL/kg)
Correct Acidosis & Hypothermia

Transfusion Targets
Hb:	80 – 100 g/L
Platelets:	>75 x 10^9/L
PT/PTT :	<1.5x normal
Fibrinogen:	>1.5 g/L
Ionised Ca^{2+}:	>1 mmol/L

Reassess
Enquire about available blood results but DO NOT WAIT for results before transfusing

Suspected continued haemorrhage: Collect & Transfuse Pack 2

Send repeat samples (including ABG, K^+, Ca^{2+})

Transfusion Packs

Pack 1
Red Cells   20 mL/kg
(Group specific if possible or O Rh D negative)

Pack 2
Red Cells   40 mL/kg
FFP   15 mL/kg
Platelets   15 mL/kg
Cryoprecipitate   15 mL/kg

Pack 3
Red Cells   40 mL/kg
FFP   15 mL/kg
Platelets   15 mL/kg
Cryoprecipitate   15 mL/kg

Patient Still Bleeding?
Send for Transfusion Pack 3
Liaise with Consultant Haematologist

Reassess
Check available blood results

Suspected continued haemorrhage: Transfuse Pack 3

Discuss with Consultant Haematologist

Further components require authorisation from Consultant Haematologist

TRAUMA

MANAGEMENT OF TRAUMATIC BRAIN INJURY (1)

Indicators of severe/time critical injury

- GCS <9
- Falling GCS
- Focal neurological deficit
- Single dilated pupil
- Depressed/open skull fracture
- CSF leak

Other indications for intubation

- Loss of protective laryngeal reflexes
- Ventilatory insufficiency:
  - hypoxaemia (PaO_2 < 9 kPa in air or < 13 kPa in O_2)

  OR
  - hypercarbia ($PaCO_2$ > 6 kPa)
- Spontaneous hyperventilation ($PaCO_2$ < 4 kPa)
- Respiratory irregularity

Children's Glasgow Coma Scale (< 4 years)		Glasgow Coma Scale (4 – 15 years)	
Response	Score	Response	Score
Eye opening		*Eye opening*	
Spontaneously	4	Spontaneously	4
To verbal stimuli	3	To verbal stimuli	3
To pain	2	To pain	2
No response to pain	1	No response to pain	1
Best verbal/non-verbal response		*Best verbal response*	
Alert; babbles, coos words to usual ability Smiles, fixes & follows	5	Orientated and converses	5
Less than usual words, spontaneous irritable cry, consolable	4	Disorientated and converses	4
Cries only to pain, inconsolable	3	Inappropriate words	3
Moans to pain. Restless/agitated	2	Incomprehensible sounds	2
No response to pain	1	No response to pain	1
Best motor response		*Best motor response*	
Spontaneous or obeys verbal command	6	Obeys verbal command	6
Localises to pain or withdraws to touch	5	Localises to pain	5
Withdraws from pain	4	Withdraws from pain	4
Abnormal flexion to pain (decorticate)	3	Abnormal flexion to pain (decorticate)	3
Abnormal extension to pain (decerebrate)	2	Abnormal extension to pain (decerebrate)	2
No response to pain	1	No response to pain	1

MANAGEMENT OF TRAUMATIC BRAIN INJURY (2)

Airway & Breathing	• Intubate and ventilate • Oral ETT, secured with tape • Aim for: **PaCO₂ 4.5 – 5.0 kPa** **PaO₂ ≥ 13 kPa** • C-spine immobilisation if suspected injury
Circulation	• Aim for: **Systolic ≥ 80 + (Age x 2) mmHg** • Adequate intravenous crystalloid resuscitation • Continue maintenance fluids • Noradrenaline if euvolaemic and **CPP < (45 + Age) mmHg**
Disability & Exposure	• 15 minute neuro observations • Sedate with Morphine and Midazolam to complete unresponsiveness to noxious stimuli (see infusions below) • Maintain paralysis while transferring patient • Treat seizures with **Phenytoin 20 mg/kg over 20 min** (Phenobarbitone in neonates) • Discuss strategy for managing raised ICP with neurosurgeons (in an emergency consider **Mannitol 0.25 – 0.5 g/kg**) • Keep 36 – 37°C, cool if needed. Warm no faster than 0.5°C/hr
On-going Management	• Head up position 15 – 30° • ICP < 20 mmHg • CPP > (45 + age) mmHg • Blood glucose 6 – 8 mmol/L • Serum sodium 140 – 150 mmol/L • HB > 100 g/L

Drug	Bolus dose	Dilution for infusion	Infusion rate
Morphine	0.1 mg/kg	1 mg/kg in 50 mL	10 – 40 microgram/kg/hr (1 mL/hr = 20 microgram/kg/hr)
Midazolam	0.1 mg/kg	6 mg/kg in 50 mL	60 – 240 microgram/kg/hr (1 mL/hr = 120 microgram/kg/hr)
Atracurium	0.5 mg/kg	Neat (10 mg/mL)	300 – 600 microgram/kg/hr (1 mL/hr = (10,000/wt in kg) microgram/kg/hr)
Rocuronium	0.6 mg/kg	Neat (10 mg/mL)	300 – 1000 microgram/kg/hr (1 mL/hr = (10,000/wt in kg) microgram/kg/hr)
Noradrenaline / Adrenaline	N/A	0.3 mg/kg in 50mL of 5% Dextrose	0.01 – 0.5 microgram/kg/min (1 mL/hr = 0.1 microgram/kg/min)

MANAGEMENT OF BURNS

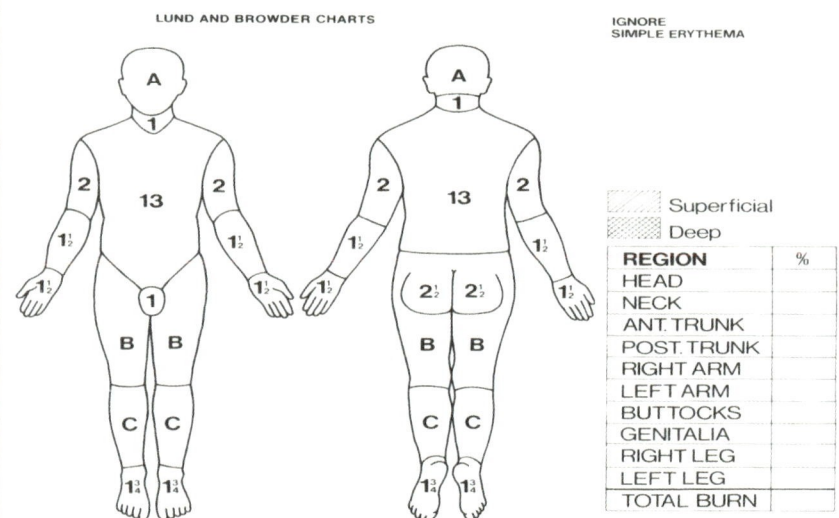

RELATIVE PERCENTAGE OF BODY SURFACE AREA AFFECTED BY GROWTH

AREA	AGE 0	1	5	10	15	ADULT
A = ½ OF HEAD	9½	8½	6½	5½	4½	3½
B = ½ OF ONE THIGH	2¾	3¼	4	4½	4½	4¾
C = ½ OF ONE LEG	2½	2½	2¾	3	3¼	3½

A I R W A Y	Indications for intubation • Airway burns • Inhalational injury • Reduced or fluctuating conscious level GCS ≤ 8	When indicated:- ➢ **Don't delay, get senior help** ➢ Intubate with oral tubes (ideally cuffed) ➢ **DON'T cut the ETT** ➢ 100% oxygen until CO levels < 10%
F L U I D S	**Parkland formula** **(Hartmann's solution)**	4 mL/kg/% BSA ➢ ½ in first 8 hr ➢ ½ in next 16 hr
	PLUS Maintenance fluids (0.9% Saline/5% Dextrose) ➢ 4:2:1 rule	Aim for **urine output > 1 mL/kg/hr** Treat shock with fluid boluses
O T H E R	• Manage as trauma (consider C-spine & secondary survey) • Check carboxyhaemoglobin levels (normal < 5%) • Access – 2 x large bore IV or IO • Analgesia – Paracetamol/opiates/Ketamine as indicated • Insert NG tube	Indications for transfer to a Burns Centre: ➢ Ventilated patients ➢ Burn area > 30% BSA ➢ Burn with poly-trauma

RADIOLOGY INFORMATION (1)

Trauma CT Guideline

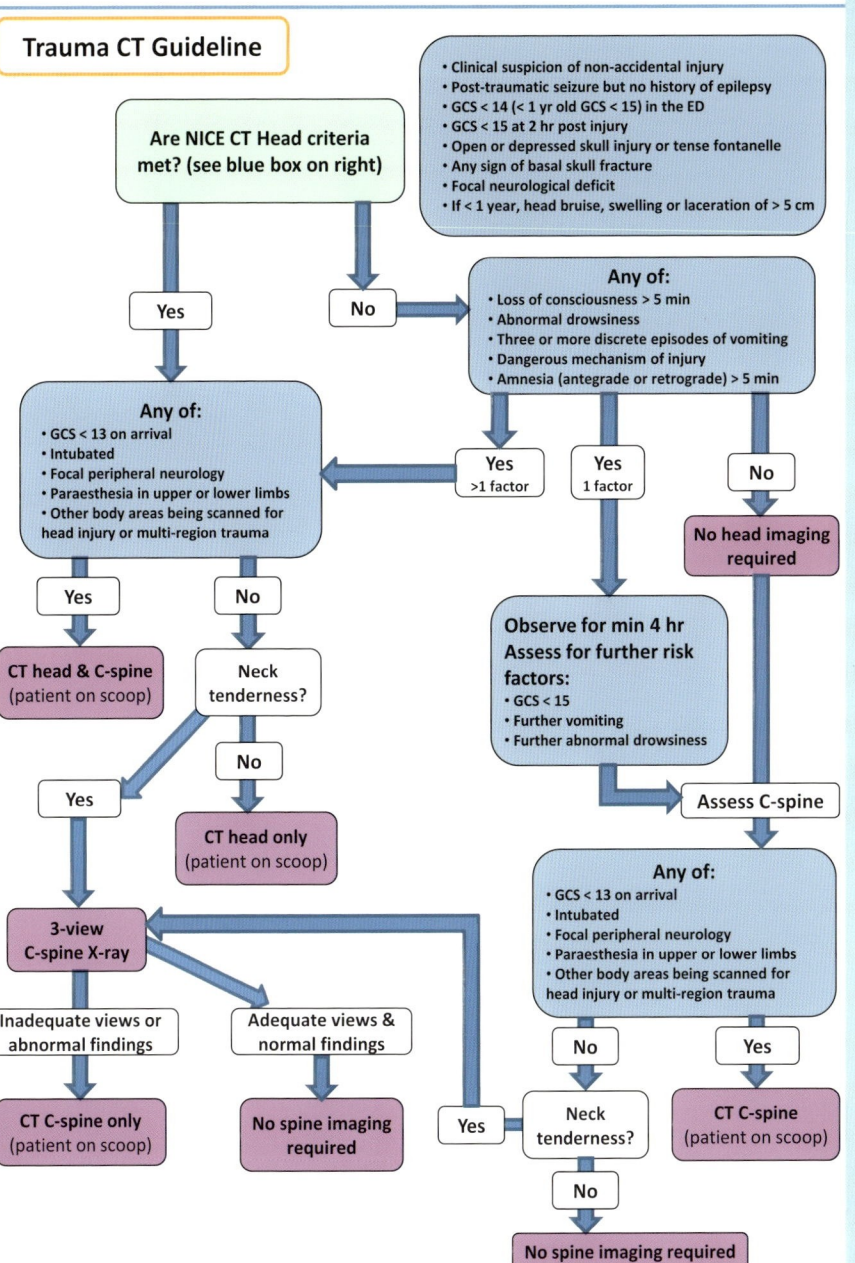

RADIOLOGY INFORMATION (2)

Abdominal CT Guideline

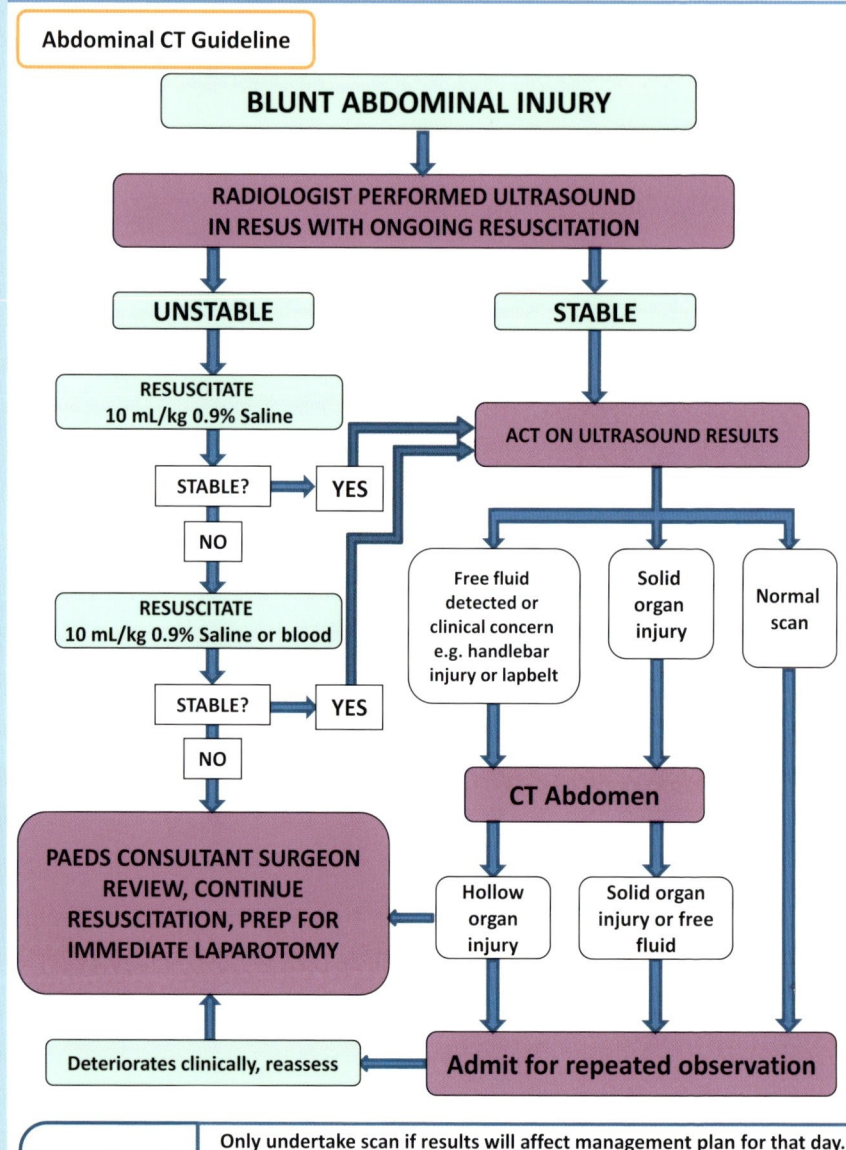

Urgent MRI Guidelines

Only undertake scan if results will affect management plan for that day.
Contraindications (D/W Consultant if emergency):
- FiO_2 > 50%
- PEEP ≥ 8
- Unstable cardiovascular status
- More than 1 inotrope infusion

UNANTICIPATED DIFFICULT MASK VENTILATION

Recognition	• Inability to maintain ventilation using face mask • Give 100% oxygen • **CALL for HELP**
Immediate management	• **Optimise head position** – chin lift/jaw thrust, shoulder roll, neutral head position, adjust/remove cricoid pressure, 2 person BMV • **Check equipment** – circuit, mask, connectors, consider using a self-inflating bag • **Increase depth of anaesthesia** – propofol 1st line • Consider CPAP

2nd stage management	• Insert oropharyngeal airway
	• **Treat cause** e.g.
	   ➢ Light anaesthesia – deepen anaesthesia
	   ➢ Laryngospasm – PEEP
	   ➢ Gastric distension – NG tube
	• **Maintain anaesthesia**
	   ➢ If paralysed, attempt intubation
	• If intubation unsuccessful, proceed to failed intubation algorithm

3rd stage management	- Insert supra-glottic airway device (LMA) ➢ **not more than 3 attempts** - Consider nasopharyngeal airway

	Good airway	**Poor airway**
3rd stage management	• Continue with procedure	• SaO_2 > 80% – consider: adjusting/changing LMA, bronchospasm/pneumothorax • SaO_2 < 80% – attempt intubation ➢ Successful – continue ➢ Unsuccessful – **proceed to failed intubation algorithm**

UNANTICIPATED DIFFICULT TRACHEAL INTUBATION

Recognition	• Difficult direct laryngoscopy • Satisfactory mask ventilation & oxygenation • Give 100% oxygen & maintain anaesthesia (CPAP & avoid gastric distension) • CALL for HELP
Immediate management	• Direct laryngoscopy – Not > 4 attempts • **Optimise head position** & laryngoscopy technique (consider: using bougie, changing blade/ETT size) • **Remove/adjust laryngeal manipulation/cricoid pressure** • **Consider inadequate paralysis** • **If intubation successful confirm position with $ETCO_2$ & auscultation** ➢ If in doubt – Remove ET tube

2nd stage management	FAILED INTUBATION with good oxygenation/mask ventilation:
	  ➢ **CALL for HELP if not arrived**
	  ➢ **Insert supra-glottic airway device (SAD) e.g. LMA; 3 attempts max**
	  ➢ **Consider use of indirect laryngoscope if experienced in use & available**

	Successful airway with SAD – consider safety of proceeding with surgery • Safe – proceed with surgery • Unsafe – postpone surgery & wake patient up • If safe – consider 1 attempt of FOI via SAD

	Failed oxygenation SaO_2 < 90% with FiO_2 1.0
	• Convert back to MV, optimise positioning, oxygenate & ventilate, apply CPAP, consider 2 person BMV, manage gastric distension, reverse non-depolarising muscle relaxant
	  ➢ **Successful – postpone surgery & wake up**
	  ➢ **Unsuccessful – proceed to "can't intubate can't ventilate" algorithm**

ANAESTHETIC

CAN'T INTUBATE, CAN'T VENTILATE (CICV)

Recognition	• Failed intubation & inadequate ventilation • Give 100% oxygen • **CALL for HELP**
Immediate management	• FiO_2 1.0, continue to attempt oxygenation & ventilation • Optimise head position – chin lift/jaw thrust • Insert oropharyngeal airway or SAD • Ventilate with a 2 person BM technique • Insert NG tube, if time permits (prevent gastric distension)
2nd stage management	➤ **Wake patient up if SaO_2 > 80%** • Reverse with suggamadex (16 mg/kg) if rocuronium/vecuronium used • Prepare for rescue techniques if patient deteriorates

3rd stage management **(Airway Rescue Techniques)**	➤ **SaO_2 < 80% & falling +/- heart rate falling:**	
	Specialist ENT support available: • Surgical tracheostomy • Rigid bronchoscopy & ventilate	**ENT unavailable:** • Percutaneous cannula cricothyroidotomy/transtracheal jet ventilation (pressure limited) ➤ Successful – continue at lowest pressure settings until wake up or definitive airway established ➤ Fail – perform surgical cricothyroidotomy/transtracheal & insertion of ETT/tracheostomy tube

<u>Cannula cricothyroidotomy</u>

- Extend neck (roll under shoulders), stabilise larynx with non-dominant hand, access cricothyroid membrane with a 14/16G cannula aimed in a caudal direction, confirm position by aspiration of air into saline-filled syringe
- Connect to either adjustable pressure limiting device set to lowest pressure OR O_2 flowmeter (flow (L/min) = child's age in yr) and a 3-way tap
- Cautiously increase inflation pressure/flow rate to achieve adequate chest expansion. Wait for full expiration before next inflation & maintain upper airway patency to aid expiration

MANAGEMENT OF MALIGNANT HYPERTHERMIA

Diagnosis & Recognition	- Unexplained increase in EtCO$_2$ with tachypnoea **AND** - Unexplained tachycardia in non-paralysed patient **AND** - Unexplained increase in oxygen requirement - Raised temperature often a **late** sign **Previous uneventful anaesthesia does not rule out MH**
Immediate management	- STOP all trigger agents - Call for help - Get MH box - Install clean breathing system & **hyperventilate with 100% O$_2$** high flow - Maintain anaesthesia with IV propofol - Muscle relaxation (Non-depolarising agent) - **Abandon/finish surgery ASAP**
Monitoring & treatment	- Give **Dantrolene** →　　**DANTROLENE** - Active cooling **Treat:** - Hyperkalaemia - Arrhythmias - Metabolic acidosis - Myoglobinuria - DIC **Bloods:** - CK - ABG - U&E's & FBC - Coagulation **DANTROLENE** **2.5 mg/kg bolus** (Mix 20 mg in 60 mL → 7.5 mL/kg) Then: **1 mg/kg repeat boluses up to 10 mg/kg** Mix vials with **water for injection** **Monitoring** - Core & peripheral temperature - EtCO$_2$, SpO$_2$, ECG - Arterial BP & CVP
Follow up	- Transfer to Paediatric ICU - Repeat Dantrolene as required - Repeat CK - Refer to MH unit at St James's Hospital, Leeds (**0113 206 5270. Emergency Hotline: 07947 609601**)

IV DANTROLENE DOSING FOR MH

WEIGHT (Kg)	1st BOLUS (mix 20 mg in 60 mL water for injection) 2.5 mg/kg = 7.5 mL/kg	Additional BOLUS 1 mg/kg = 3 mL/kg	Maximum cumulative dose 10 mg/kg = 30 ml/kg
1	7.5 mL	3 mL	30 mL
5	37.5 mL	15 mL	150 mL
10	75.0 mL	30 mL	300 mL
15	112.5 mL	45 mL	450 mL
20	150.0 mL	60 mL	600 mL
25	187.5 mL	75 mL	750 mL
30	225.0 mL	90 mL	900 mL
35	262.5 mL	105 mL	1050 mL
40	300.0 mL	120 mL	1200 mL
45	337.5 mL	135 mL	1350 mL
50	375.0 mL	150 mL	1500 mL
55	412.5 mL	165 mL	1650 mL
60	450.0 mL	180 mL	1800 mL
65	487.5 mL	195 mL	1950 mL
70	525.0 mL	210 mL	2100 mL

Remember to include Dantrolene solution volume in child's total fluid balance record

MANAGEMENT OF SEVERE LOCAL ANAESTHETIC TOXICITY

Diagnosis & Recognition	**CNS:** Sudden alteration in mental state or loss of consciousness with or without seizures **CVS:** Cardiovascular collapse; conduction blocks, sinus bradycardia, asystole and ventricular tachyarrhythmia **These may occur some time after injection**
Immediate management	• Stop injection of local anaesthetic • **Call for help** • Give 100% oxygen and ensure adequate lung ventilation • Confirm/establish venous access • Control of seizures: give **benzodiazepine** or **thiopentone** or **propofol** in small incremental doses • Monitor cardiovascular status throughout
Local Anaesthetic-induced Cardiac Arrest Management	• **Start cardiopulmonary resuscitation** as per protocol • Manage arrhythmias as APLS protocol: may be refractory to standard treatment • Prolonged resuscitation may be necessary • **Consider treatment with lipid emulsion** (See Page 39): 1. Give an intravenous bolus injection of **intralipid 20% 1.5 mL/kg** over 1 min 2. Follow immediately with an **infusion rate of 15 mL/kg/hr** 3. Continue **CPR** to circulate intralipid 4. Repeat bolus 1 – 2 times at 5 min interval, if inadequate circulation persists 5. After another 5 min increase the rate to 30 mL/kg/hr if cardiovascular stability is not restored or an adequate circulation deteriorates 6. Continue infusion until CVS stability or max. dose of intralipid is given 7. Review infusion rate every 15 – 20 min, reduce & stop when clinical parameters allow **A maximum total dose of 12 mL/kg is recommended**
Follow up	Report all cases to National Patient Safety Agency and to the Lipid Rescue site: www.npsa.nhs.uk & www.lipidrescue.org If possible take blood samples into a plain tube (red top) & a heparinized tube (green top) before and after lipid emulsion. Measure lipid and local anaesthetic levels

IV INTRALIPID 20% DOSING FOR LOCAL ANAESTHETIC-INDUCED CARDIAC ARREST

WEIGHT (Kg)	BOLUS Intralipid 20% 1.5 mL/kg IV over 1 minute	INFUSION Start at: 15 mL/kg/hr	INFUSION Increase to 30 mL/kg/hr if inadequate circulation persists	Maximum cumulative dose 12 mL/kg
1	1.5 mL	15 mL/hr	30 mL/hr	12 mL
2	3.0 mL	30 mL/hr	60 mL/hr	24 mL
3	4.5 mL	45 mL/hr	90 mL/hr	36 mL
4	6.0 mL	60 mL/hr	120 mL/hr	48 mL
5	7.5 mL	75 mL/hr	150 mL/hr	60 mL
6	9.0 mL	90 mL/hr	180 mL/hr	72 mL
7	10.5 mL	105 mL/hr	210 mL/hr	84 mL
8	12.0 mL	120 mL/hr	240 mL/hr	96 mL
9	13.5 mL	135 mL/hr	270 mL/hr	108 mL
10	15.0 mL	150 mL/hr	300 mL/hr	120 mL
15	22.5 mL	225 mL/hr	450 mL/hr	180 mL
20	30.0 mL	300 mL/hr	600 mL/hr	240 mL
25	37.5 mL	375 mL/hr	750 mL/hr	300 mL
30	45.0 mL	450 mL/hr	900 mL/hr	360 mL
35	52.5 mL	525 mL/hr	1050 mL/hr	420 mL
40	60.0 mL	600 mL/hr	1200 mL/hr	480 mL
45	67.5 mL	675 mL/hr	1350 mL/hr	540 mL
50	75.0 mL	750 mL/hr	1500 mL/hr	600 mL
55	82.5 mL	825 mL/hr	1650 mL/hr	660 mL
60	90.0 mL	900 mL/hr	1800 mL/hr	720 mL
70	100 mL	1000 mL/hr	2000 mL/hr	840 mL
80	120 mL	1200 mL/hr	2400 mL/hr	960 mL
90	135 mL	1350 mL/hr	2700 mL/hr	1080 mL
100	150 mL	1500 mL/hr	3000 mL/hr	1200 mL

PAEDIATRIC PAIN GUIDELINES (1)

MORPHINE

N.C.A. NEONATAL up to 12 wks
Drug concentration = 10 microgram/kg/mL
i.e. 0.5 mg morphine/kg/bodyweight diluted to 50 mL with 0.9% Saline

PUMP PROGRAMME
- Loading dose = zero
- Bolus dose = 0.5 mL
- Lockout = 60 min
- Background infusion = 0.5 – 1 mL/hr

N.C.A. INFANT – 13 wks to 6 months
Drug concentration = 10 microgram/kg/mL
i.e. 0.5 mg morphine/kg/bodyweight diluted to 50 mL with 0.9% Saline

PUMP PROGRAMME
- Loading dose = zero
- Bolus dose = 1 mL
- Lockout = 30 min
- Background infusion = 1 mL/hr

N.C.A. CHILDREN from 6 months
Drug concentration = 20 microgram/kg/mL
i.e. 1 mg morphine/kg/bodyweight (max. 50 mg) diluted to 50 mL with 0.9% Saline

PUMP PROGRAMME
- Loading dose = zero
- Bolus dose = 1 mL
- Lockout = 30 min
- Background infusion = 1 mL/hr

P.C.A. CHILDREN > 6 YEARS
i.e. 1 mg morphine/kg/bodyweight (max. 50 mg) diluted to 50 mL with 0.9% Saline

PUMP PROGRAMME
- Loading dose = zero
- Bolus dose = 1 mL
- Lockout = 5 min
- Background infusion = 0.2 mL/hr

ORAL MORPHINE

AGE	DOSE	INTERVAL
< 3/12	50 microgram/kg	6 hourly
3/12 – 6/12	50 – 100 microgram/kg	4 hourly
6/12 – 1 yr	100 microgram/kg	4 hourly
1 yr – 2 yr	200 – 400 microgram/kg	4 hourly
> 2 yr	200 – 500 microgram/kg	4 hourly

Use lower end of dose range if using as codeine replacement

FENTANYL

To be used for renal patients requiring post-operative intravenous opiates

OR

Patients with inadequate analgesia with morphine

N.C.A. CHILDREN from 13 WEEKS
Drug concentration = 1 microgram/kg/mL
i.e. 50 microgram/kg bodyweight (max. 2500 microgram) = 1 mL NEAT fentanyl/kg bodyweight – diluted to 50 mL with 0.9% Saline

PUMP PROGRAMME
- Loading dose = zero
- Bolus dose = 1 mL
- Lockout = 30 min
- Background infusion = 1 mL/hr

P.C.A. CHILDREN > 6 YEARS
Drug concentration = 1 microgram/kg/mL
i.e. 50 microgram/kg bodyweight (max. 2500 microgram) = 1 mL NEAT fentanyl/kg bodyweight – diluted to 50 mL with 0.9% Saline

PUMP PROGRAMME
- Loading dose = zero
- Bolus dose = 0.5 mL
- Lockout = 6 – 10 min
- Background infusion = 0.5 mL/hr

KETAMINE

Drug concentration = 40 microgram/kg/mL
i.e. 2 mg Ketamine/kg bodyweight (max. 100 mg) diluted to 50 mL with 0.9% Saline

PCA
Indications : Pancolitis & risk of toxic megacolon
- Loading dose = 1 – 2 mL of solution
- Infusion 0 – 1 mL/hr
- Bolus 0.5 – 1 mL
- Lockout 10 – 30 min

Infusion
Indications – scoliosis surgery or complex analgesia requirements
- Loading dose = 1 – 2 mL of solution
- Infusion 0 – 5 mL/hr

Must be discussed with a Consultant Anaesthetist

PAEDIATRIC PAIN GUIDELINES (2)

LOCAL ANAESTHETICS

EPIDURAL CHILDREN > 13 wks

Drugs & concentration = 0.1% Levo-bupivacaine
+ Fentanyl 2 microgram/mL

OR   Plain 0.125% Levo-bupivacaine

Rate = 0.1 – 0.3 mL/kg/hr   (maximum 15 mL/hr)

EPIDURAL TROUBLE SHOOTING

1. Block but inadequate analgesia: Increase rate within prescribed range OR change to plain L-bupivacaine plus NCA/PCA

2. Inadequate/no block: Bolus 0.1 mL/kg of 0.25% L – bupivacaine, assess BP every 5 min for 15 min

3. If NO improvement in block: Change to NCA/PCA

Boluses – ONLY by members of anaesthetic department or pain service

REGIONAL BLOCK & WOUND CATHETERS

Drug & concentration = 0.125% L-bupivacaine

Wound catheter infusions
Child 0 – 8 years   - rate 0 – 2 mL/hr
Child 9 years and over - rate 0 – 5 mL/hr

Paravertebral
Rate = 0 – 0.2 mL/kg/hr   (maximum = 10 mL/hr)

Caudal analgesia
Drug & concentration = 0.25% L-bupivacaine
Volume = 0.5 – 1.0 mL/kg single shot
Possible caudal additives:
- Preservative-free S-ketamine: 0.5 mg/kg
  (for children > 12 months of age)
- Clonidine: 1 microgram/kg

OTHER DRUGS

ANTIEMETICS

ONDANSETRON
0.15 mg/kg 8 hourly IV or PO   **Max = 4 mg**

DEXAMETHASONE
0.15 mg/kg 8 hourly IV or PO   **Max = 4 mg**

ANALGESICS

PARACETAMOL – PO
Under 13 weeks: loading dose 20 mg/kg then 20 mg/kg TDS. **Max 60 mg/kg daily**
Over 13 weeks: loading dose 20 mg/kg then 15 mg/kg QDS. **Max 90 mg/kg or 4 g daily**

PARACETAMOL – INTRAVENOUS
Preterm > 32 weeks: 7.5 mg/kg TDS. **Max 25 mg/kg daily**
Neonate: 10 mg/kg TDS. **Max 30 mg/kg daily**
Child body weight <50 kg: 15 mg/kg 4 hourly. **Max 60 mg/kg daily**
Child body weight >50 kg: 1 g 4 hourly. **Max 4 g daily**

IBUPROFEN (NSAID)
<5 kg weight = **Not recommended**
Child over 5 kg body weight: 5 mg/kg QDS
(10 mg/kg severe pain)   **Max 2.4 g daily**

DICLOFENAC (NSAID)
<6 mths (postoperative pain)   - **Not recommended**
From 6 mths   - 1 mg/kg TDS
Max. daily dose = 150 mg for children >50 kg

NALOXONE – IV OR IM
4 microgram/kg – stat dose   **Max 200 microgram**
(always prescribe with NCA/PCA)

CHLORPHENAMINE/PIRITON
0.1 mg/kg 8 hourly. **Max 4 mg (PO) or 5 mg (IV)**

1st choice for treatment of opiate-induced itch is Ondansetron.
Piriton may cause excessive drowsiness with opiates

FLUID MANAGEMENT (1)

Aim of peri-operative fluids is to replace deficit (starvation/dehydration), provide ongoing maintenance requirements & replace intra-operative losses (3rd space/blood loss)

Maintenance fluids
• **NPSA alert 2007** – Only isotonic solutions should be used as maintenance fluids. Hypotonic solutions may result in hyponatraemia due to retention of free water released after metabolism of dextrose. Children are also prone to exhibiting syndrome of inappropriate anti-diuretic secretion (SIADH) in response to pain, nausea/vomiting, pyrexia, sepsis, head injury

Pre- and post-operatively
• Appropriate fluid is the isotonic solution: 0.9% saline/5% Dextrose
• Children receiving IV fluids should have daily urea and electrolytes measured and ideally have their weight checked daily.
• Post-operatively either give full maintenance OR restrict to 60 – 70% of maintenance plus boluses of isotonic solutions as required to maintain urine output.

Intra-operatively
• The risk of hypoglycaemia developing in healthy children is unusual as blood glucose tends to increase due to the stress response to surgery.
• Children at risk of hypoglycaemia include: Neonates
                                                Those on TPN
                                                Those with extensive regional analgesia techniques
• These patients should have their blood glucose recorded intra-operatively.
• Neonates should receive 10% Dextrose with added sodium chloride and those on TPN should have this continued intra-operatively.
• The majority of children do not required Dextrose-containing solutions intra-operatively and Ringer's lactate/Hartmann's solution or 0.9% saline are appropriate solutions.

Formula:

Formula	Body weight 1st 10 kg (0 – 10 kg)	Body weight 11 – 20 kg	Body weight > 20 kg	Total
Holiday & Segar derived formula	100 mL/kg/day	1000 mL + 50 mL/kg/day For 2nd 10 kg	1500 mL + 20 mL/kg/day For all kg over 20 kg	mL per 24 hours
4:2:1 formula	4 mL/kg/hr	40 mL + 2 mL/kg/hr for 2nd 10 kg	60 mL + 1 mL/kg/hr for all kg over 20 kg	mL per hour

FLUID MANAGEMENT (2)

Correction of fluid deficit
- Minimise fluid deprivation period – safe to have clear fluids up to 2 hours before surgery.
- Fasting deficit = number of hours fluids restricted x hourly maintenance . Replace 50% in 1st hour & 25% in 2nd & 3rd hours (Furman *et al* 1975)
- Assessment of dehydration from clinical signs is inaccurate. Best method uses difference between current weight and accurate pre-morbid weight
- **Correction of 1% dehydration requires 10 mL/kg of fluid**
- Ringers lactate or 0.9% saline are appropriate fluids

Third space losses
- Replace with Ringers lactate or 0.9% saline
- Vary with procedure:
    - 1 – 2 mL/kg/hr   Peripheral & neurosurgery
    - 4 – 7 mL/kg/hr   Thoracic surgery
    - 6 – 10 mL/kg/hr   Abdominal surgery
    - Up to 50 mL/kg   NEC surgery
- Replace NG/stoma losses with 0.9% saline

Blood loss
- Decision made on concept of an allowable blood loss (ABL) and estimated blood volume (EBV):
    - **EBV: Neonate 80 – 90 mL/kg; Infant 80 mL/kg; Child 75 – 80 mL/kg; Adult 70 mL/kg**
    - **ABL = EBV x (Hb $_{(start)}$ – Hb $_{(lowest\ acceptable)}$)/Hb $_{(start)}$**
- Replace blood loss with crystalloid (ratio 3:1) or colloid (ratio 1:1) until transfusion limit reached

Treatment of hyponatraemia – Na^+ <135 mmol/L
- Early signs are non-specific. Often presents with seizures or respiratory arrest.
- First line treatment is an infusion of 3% saline until seizures stop or Na^+ >125 mmol/L (1 mL/kg will raise the Na^+ by 1 mmol/L)
- Mmol of Na^+ required = (130 – present Na^+) x 0.6 x wt (kg)
- Once Na^+ > 125 mmol/L then correction can be slower and fluid changed to 0.9% saline
- The asymptomatic child with a normal or increased fluid status should have their oral or IV maintenance fluids reduced to 50%

Treatment of hypernatraemia – Na^+ >150 mmol/L
- Develops due to restricted water intake, inability to respond to thirst, excessive water loss or inappropriately made up infant feeds. Symptoms are more severe when hypernatraemia develops rapidly, chronic hypernatraemia is generally well tolerated
- The degree of dehydration is often underestimated as circulating volume is maintained at the expense of intracellular water
- Initial management involves a 20 mL/kg bolus of 0.9% saline to restore circulating volume
- Further correction should be done over 48 hours to prevent development of cerebral oedema. Serum Na^+ should not increase by more than 12 mmol/L/day. Maintenance fluids must be run along-side correction fluids

CONGENITAL CARDIAC DISEASE

- Most common birth defect (1 : 125 live births). > 90% survive to adulthood
- Present with the same elective & emergency conditions as other children
- In general, ↑ risk of morbidity, cardiac events and 30-day mortality

Normal Circulation with Shunt

e.g. ASD, VSD, PDA
- Blood flows down pressure gradient:
  - L > R : ↑ Pulmonary flow (PBF) & ↓ systemic flow => systemic acidosis
  - R > L : ↓ PBF & cyanosis
- ➢ Ensure adequate fluid loading (avoid long starvation)
- ➢ Minimise disruption to SVR:PVR ratio

Persistent Parallel Circulation

e.g. Hypoplastic left heart, Complete AVSD
- Pulmonary & systemic circulations freely communicate
- Blood flow dependent on relative resistances in systemic & pulmonary circulations (SVR & PVR)
- ➢ Best managed in specialist centre
- ➢ Monitor pre- and post- shunt & maintain preload
- ➢ Maintain SVR:PVR ratio:
  - ➢ SVR : ↓with anaesthetics & ↑ with inotropes
  - ➢ PVR : ↑ - ↓PaO_2, ↑$PaCO_2$, Nitrous Oxide
    ↓ - ↑PaO_2, ↓$PaCO_2$, pharmacology

Surgical Palliation (Single Ventricle)

Multi-stage generation of 'in series' circulation
- Ventricle supplies systemic circulation; pulmonary blood flow is via passive systemic venous return

Stage 1 (BT Shunt)
- ➢ **Most difficult to manage**
- ➢ Balance between SVR & PVR **CRITICAL**
- ➢ Maintain normal/high CO_2 & low FiO_2
- ➢ Monitor SpO_2 (70 – 80%) & lactate

Stage 2 (Glenn Shunt)
- ➢ SpO_2 in mid-80s
- ➢ Aim to reduce load on RV
- ➢ Often chronically cyanosed & polycythaemic
- ➢ Maintain preload & avoid hypovolaemia

Stage 3 (Fontan Circulation)
- ➢ SpO_2 usually normal, ↓ if PVR increases
- ➢ Essential that PVR remains low
- ➢ Maintain hydration & avoid ventilation if possible
- ➢ Careful ventilation in long cases (see below)

GENERAL ANAESTHETIC CONSIDERATIONS

INDUCTION:
- IV: Propofol : ↓↓SVR & MAP, ↑Right-to-Left shunt ⇒ ↓ SpO_2
  Ketamine : Minimal effect on SVR, PVR or MAP. Best agent in Pulmonary Hypertension
- Inhalational : Common choice, avoid prolonged 8% sevoflurane

MAINTENANCE:
- Isoflurane/Sevoflurane : Minimal effect on myocardial contractility or shunt fraction
- Avoid propofol

ANALGESIA:
- Fentanyl (+/- infusion) or regional techniques

OXYGEN:
- High FiO_2: ↓PVR; can ↑ Left-to-Right shunt ⇒ ↓systemic perfusion & pulmonary oedema

VENTILATION:
- Consider spontaneous ventilation to aid pulmonary blood flow
- **MUST avoid:** hypoxia, hypercarbia & atelectasis (which ↑PVR & ↓PBF)
- If ventilating, **avoid**: High pressures; high PEEP & long inspiratory times

OTHER:
- Slight head-up & raising legs aids venous return & PBF
- Extreme care to avoid air bubbles in lines

CCD FOR NON-CARDIAC SURGERY

- Children with CCD presenting for non-cardiac surgery are at increased risk
- Range of heart disease & variety of procedures make this hard to quantify
- Most important factors:

1) Physiological Status:

- **Cardiac Failure** (Very high risk)
  - Signs differ with age
  - Tachypnoea, tachycardia, sweating & cool peripheries
- **Pulmonary Hypertension**
  - PAP >25 mmHg at rest (or 30 mmHg on exercise)
  - Clear predictor of morbidity
- **Arrhythmias**
- **Cyanosis**
  - Common in unrepaired or partially palliated
  - Chronic cyanosis affects most organ systems
  - Polycythaemia & coagulopathy main problem
  - Dehydration, fever & anaemia MUST be avoided

2) Complexity of Heart Disease:

Considered 'complex' if any of:
- Single ventricle physiology
- Parallel circulation physiology
- Cardiomyopathy
- Aortic stenosis

3) Type of Operation:

- Major vs. Minor
- Elective vs. Emergency
- Risk of blood loss
- Prolonged hospital stay

RISK CLASSIFICATION:

HIGH RISK	INTERMEDIATE RISK	LOW RISK
Physiologically poorly compensated +/- presence of major complications: ➢ Cardiac Failure ➢ Pulmonary Hypertension ➢ Arrhythmias ➢ Cyanosis	Physiologically normal or well compensated	Physiologically normal or well compensated
Complex lesions	Simple lesions	Simple lesions
Major surgery (intra-peritoneal, intra-thoracic or anticipated major blood loss)	Major surgery (intra-peritoneal, intra-thoracic or anticipated major blood loss)	Minor (or body surface) surgery
Under 2 years	Under 2 years	Over 2 years
Emergency	Emergency	Elective
Pre-op hospital stay > 10 days	Pre-op hospital stay > 10 days	Pre-op hospital stay < 10 days
ASA IV or V	ASA IV or V	ASA I – III

SUGGESTED MANAGEMENT:

RISK	ELECTIVE	EMERGENCY
High	Transfer to specialist centre	➢ Seek advice from PICU & surgeons about possibility of transfer ➢ If impossible: advice from cardiologist & cardiac anaesthetist re: peri-op management ➢ Transfer post-op as soon as stable
Intermediate	Discuss with specialist centre and consider transfer	
Low	Manage at local hospital	Manage locally If concerned, seek advice

COMMON SYNDROMES & CONGENITAL CONDITIONS (1)

Syndrome	Description	Clinical features	Anaesthetic considerations
Achondroplasia	Commonest form of dwarfism. 1/25,000 live births Defective fibroblast growth factor 3 affecting bone formation	Shortened tubular bones Foramen magnum & spinal stenosis may occur Sleep apnoea secondary to midface hypoplasia & brainstem compression Macrocephaly Hypotonia & lax skin	Often require smaller ETT than age suggests Caution with neck movements IV access may be difficult Sleep apnoea – consider sleep studies and post-operative care
Angelman syndrome (Happy puppet syndrome)	Genetic defect in maternal chromosome 15q 1/10 – 20,000 incidence	Appear normal at birth Mental retardation, craniofacial abnormalities, drooling, ataxia, seizures, paroxysmal laughter, muscle atrophy, vagal over activity, thoracic scoliosis	Caution with GABA and NMDA receptor active drugs Inhalational technique preferable **Risk of difficult intubation** (progressive) Consider anticholinergic to overcome vagal tone
Apert syndrome	1/50,000 live births Fibroblast growth factor receptor 2 defect	Mental retardation, hypoplastic maxilla, exophthalmos, craniosynostosis, fused cervical vertebrae, narrow trachea with fused rings, congenital heart disease, 50% have raised ICP, syndactyly	**Mask ventilation may be difficult** but intubation usually easy High incidence of URTI complications. Increased incidence of bronchospasm OSA – may need post-op CPAP Eyes susceptible to damage – lubricate well
Charcot Marie Tooth (Peroneal muscular atrophy)	Hereditary polyneuropathy	Muscle weakness (limb) Cardiac problems including conduction defects, arrhythmias & cardiomyopathy Potential association with malignant hyperthermia although doubtful	Normal response to non-depolarising muscle relaxants Volatiles have been used without problem
CHARGE association	**C** – Coloboma **H** – Heart defect **A** – Atresia choanae & clefts **R** – Retarded growth & development **G** – Genital hypoplasia & renal abnormality **E** – Ear anomalies & deafness	Mid-face hypoplasia & micrognathia 75% have a congenital heart defect (commonest: Tetralogy of Fallot)	**Difficult airway and intubation with increasing difficulty as age increases** Reflux common Echo to assess CHD Abdominal US for renal anomalies

COMMON SYNDROMES & CONGENITAL CONDITIONS (2)

Syndrome	Description	Clinical features	Anaesthetic considerations
Cornelia de Lange syndrome	Approx 1:40,000	Short stature, microcephaly, facial dysmorphism, dysmorphic limbs, hirsuitism, developmental delay, cardiac & renal malformations, characteristic low pitched cry	Reflux common **Intubation may be difficult. Consider FOI** Susceptibility to malignant hyperthermia has been reported
Cri du Chat syndrome	Chromosomal abnormality (5p deletion) 1:15,000 to 1:50,000	Mental retardation, characteristic cat-like cry, microcephaly, broad nasal bridge, micrognathia, may have abnormal epiglottis and small larynx. Small incidence of congenital heart defects & renal abnormalities	Airway – Anticipate need for smaller ETT **Intubation may be difficult**
Crouzon syndrome	Chromosomal abnormality leading to premature closure of cranial sutures Progressive condition usually manifesting before the age of 2	Craniosynostosis & facial hypoplasia (especially maxilla) and exophthalmos. May lead to raised intracranial pressure	**Mask ventilation difficult but tracheal intubation usually straightforward** Post-op airway obstruction may be a problem. Airway access may be limited by external fixation devices for maxillary distraction. Eye protection important
DiGeorge syndrome (Catch 22 syndrome)	3rd and 4th brachial arch abnormalities 22q deletion	Severe cardiac malformations. Aortic arch abnormalities. Midface hypoplasia & micrognathia. Absent thymus and parathyroid glands, low serum calcium leading to tetany and seizures. Immunodeficient	**Anticipate difficult airway.** Sterile techniques required as immunodeficient. Need irradiated blood, check calcium levels & supplement. Adrenaline may cause prolonged tachycardia
Down syndrome	Trisomy 21 1 in 700 live births	Developmental delay. CCD (ASD / VSD / AVSD / PDA). Hypotonia, atlantoaxial instability (12%). Micrognathia, large tongue, congenital subglottic stenosis, tonsillar hyperplasia & OSA. Hypothyroidism	Careful airway and cardiac assessment. **Mask ventilation may be difficult.** Consider small ET tube. Care with neck extension

COMMON SYNDROMES & CONGENITAL CONDITIONS (3)

Syndrome	Description	Clinical features	Anaesthetic considerations
Edward's syndrome	Trisomy 18 1 in 8,000 live births	Mental retardation, hypotonia, renal abnormalities & CCD. Micrognathia	**May be difficult airway & intubation** Sux can cause rigidity
Ehlers-Danlos syndromes	Collagen abnormality	Hyper-elastic & fragile tissue. Dissecting aortic aneurysms. May affect clotting, heart, lung & GI	Difficult IV access Increased bleeding Spont. pneumothorax
Eisenmenger syndrome	Reversal of Left-to-Right shunt caused by pulmonary hypertension	Right-to-Left shunt Dyspnoea, fatigue, cyanosis, finger clubbing & cardiac failure	Assess cardiac function. Inhalation or SLOW IV induction. Avoid ↑ PVR (hypoxemia, hypercarbia, acidosis or N_2O) or ↓ SVR (high dose induction agents, SNP). Caution with IPPV (minimise intra-thoracic pressure) & fluid therapy (avoid hypovolaemia or over hydration)
Fanconi's syndrome	Anaemia with renal tubular acidosis	Usually due to cystinosis Impaired renal function, acidosis, K loss, dehydration. Thyroid & pancreatic dysfunction possible. May need renal transplant in 2nd decade	Correct electrolyte and acid-base abnormalities Caution with renally excreted drugs
Goldenhar syndrome	Oculoauriculovertebral syndrome; hemifacial microsomia	Unilateral mandibular hypoplasia Chromosome 22 trisomy. 20% have CHD Vertebral abnormalities may limit neck extension	**Potentially difficult airway:- BMV may be difficult. Tracheal intubation may be very difficult** especially with bilateral disease or right sided TMJ & mandible involved
Haemolytic uraemic syndrome	Renal failure, haemolytic anaemia and thrombocytopenia	Usually occurs in 1 – 2 year olds following a prodromal GI infection. CVS (hypotension, myocarditis, CCF), CNS (drowsiness, seizures, coma), respiratory-pulmonary insufficiency, hepatosplenomegaly, coagulopathy, decreased platelet function	Assessment of respiratory function Correct electrolyte, acid-base and coagulation abnormalities Caution with renally excreted drugs

COMMON SYNDROMES & CONGENITAL CONDITIONS (4)

Syndrome	Description	Clinical features	Anaesthetic considerations
Haemophilia	Factor VIII deficiency (Classic haemophilia type A) X-linked recessive, incidence 1 in 10,000	Bleeding either spontaneous or after minimal injury, haemarthrosis are common	Infusions of recombinant factor VIII 1 hr before and after surgery to maintain factor VIII activity ≥ 50%
Idiopathic thrombocytopenia	Autoimmune disease associated with presence of antiplatelet factor	Thrombocytopenia Severe GI or intracranial bleeding rare in children Chronic ITP more likely in children > 10 yr of age Treatment with high dose steroids and γ-globulin	Steroid cover many be necessary due to steroid therapy Avoid NSAIDs and IM injections
Juvenile rheumatoid arthritis	Still's disease (systemic), polyarticular or pauciarticular forms	Joint pain & stiffness, fever, rash, lymphadenopathy, uveitis	Steroid supplement required
Klippel-Feil syndrome	Congenital fusion of 2 or more cervical vertebrae	Reduced cervical mobility. Associated with Arnold-Chiari malformation & scoliosis	**Plan for a difficult intubation** due to neck immobility
Leopard syndrome	Cardio-cutaneous syndrome	Multiple large freckles, hypertelorism, deafness, CHD, progressive hypertrophic cardiomyopathy, arrhythmias, growth retardation, kyphosis, genitourinary anomalies	Assess cardiorespiratory function, monitor ECG **Intubation may be difficult**
Long QT syndrome	Jervell-Lange-Nielsen syndrome	Congenital deafness and cardiac conduction defects (arrhythmias & syncopal episodes), serious arrhythmias (VF) may occur under GA ECG shows large T waves and prolonged Q-T interval	Discuss with a cardiologist. GA may precipitate arrhythmias. Pre-treat with B blockers to decrease risk. Avoid atropine and volatiles. TIVA with propofol and remifentanil may be optimal. Treat VF with lidocaine & defibrillation
Marfan syndrome	Arachnodactyly Mutant gene on chromosome 15 causing connective tissue disorder	Tall, thin usually male patients, long fingers and face, high arched palate, joint instability including cervical spine, kyphoscoliosis, pectus excavatum, spontaneous pneumothorax (4%), aortic root dilation causing incompetence or aneurysm	Preoperative cardiac assessment required **Intubation may be difficult**. Care needed to prevent damage to C-spine or temporomandibular joint. Beware of pneumothorax Avoid hypertension

COMMON SYNDROMES & CONGENITAL CONDITIONS (5)

Syndrome	Description	Clinical features	Anaesthetic considerations
Muco-polysaccharidosis (Hurler's, Hunter's)	Abnormal mucopolysaccharide metabolism with progressive deposition in tissues	Mental retardation, gargoyle facies, deafness, stiff joints, severe coronary artery disease, hepatosplenomegaly. Most die from respiratory/cardiac failure before 10 years of age. Hunter's less severe than Hurler's	**Difficult airway management & intubation** – upper airway obstruction due to lymphoid tissue infiltration, micrognathia, short neck & limited movement of TMJ
Muscular dystrophies (Duchenne's, Becker's, facioscapulohumeral)	Inherited disorders of muscle due to abnormality/absence of the protein dystrophin. **Duchenne** – X linked recessive mutation on chromosome 21, incidence 1 in 3000 live male births. **Becker** – X linked recessive, incidence 1 in 60,000, later onset and slower progression than Duchenne. **Facioscapulohumeral muscular dystrophy** – autosomal dominant, relatively benign, slowly progressive, affects abductors of upper arms, facial muscles, winged scapula, sensorineural deafness, retinopathy	Progressive muscle weakness of affected muscle groups (pseudohypertrophied). **Duchenne** – onset between 1 – 4 years, wheelchair bound by 12 years, cardiac involvement with hypertrophic cardiomyopathy and sudden death, scoliosis, mental retardation (30%), death from cardiorespiratory failure in 3rd decade	Discus benefits vs risk. Assess cardiac function including ejection fraction, consider invasive monitoring. Respiratory function tests to help predicted need for post-op ventilation. Prone to LRTI. Regional analgesia useful. **Suxamethonium contraindicated** – risk of rhabdomyolysis, rigidity, hyperkalaemia, cardiac arrest. Variable response to non-depolarising muscle relaxants. Reduction in dose recommended. Significant myocardial depression with volatiles. NO proven link with MH but muscle damage & hyperkalaemia may occur with volatiles, hence TIVA often used. PHDU / PICU post-op
Myasthenia gravis	Juvenile/autoimmune myasthenia	Presentation in childhood or adolescence with muscle fatigability/weakness either generalized or limited to ocular muscles	Muscle weakness may cause respiratory failure. Anticholinesterases cause increased respiratory secretions. Increased sensitivity to non-depolarizing muscle relaxants – intubate deep / topical lignocaine to trachea. Avoid opiates & sedative premedication

COMMON SYNDROMES & CONGENITAL CONDITIONS (6)

Syndrome	Description	Clinical features	Anaesthetic considerations
Myopathies (Central core, nemaline myopathy, King syndrome)	Inherited diseases of muscle function **Central core disease** – autosomal dominant, gene mutation on chromosome 19 close to gene responsible for ryanidine receptor **Nemaline myopathy** – autosomal recessive & dominant inheritance, mutations on chromosome 1, 2 & 19 **King syndrome** – myopathy, MH trait, dysmorphic features (Noonan like)	**Central core** – hypotonia at birth, proximal muscle weakness, kyphoscoliosis, joint hypermobility, short neck, mandibular hypoplasia. Symptoms mild & non-progressive **Closely associated with MH** **Nemaline rod** – weakness of proximal muscles, facial, bulbar & respiratory. Dysmorphic feature (micrognathia, hypertelorism, high arched palate), cardiac abnormalities "Typical" – infantile hypotonia, non-progressive "Severe" – presents at birth with severe hypotonia, respiratory failure, arthrogryposis, death in first few months of life	**Central core disease & King syndrome** – treat **patients as MH susceptible**. Avoid all trigger agents Assess degree of muscle weakness preoperatively **Nemaline rod** – NO association with MH Prone to recurrent aspirations & LRTI Assess respiratory function & optimise with physio **Intubation may be difficult** Resistant to suxamethonium but increased sensitivity to non-depolarising muscle relaxants May need post-operative ventilation & respiratory complications are most common cause of death
Noonan syndrome	Turner's characteristics without sex chromosome abnormality	Short stature, web neck, mild mental retardation CCD (pul. stenosis & cardiomyopathy) Micrognathia, hydronephrosis & platelet dysfunction	Assess cardiac function Check coagulation & renal function **Possible difficult intubation**
Osler-Weber-Rendu syndrome	Hereditary haemorrhagic telangiectasia	Multiple skin and mucosa lesions. May affect other organs, esp. pulmonary & hepatic AV fistula Anaemia & systemic emboli. Later, high output cardiac failure	Intra-op blood loss may be difficult to control Difficult IV access Assess pulmonary function
Osteogenesis imperfecta	Pathological fractures	Fractures, blue sclera & deafness. Scoliosis & lung pathology	Extreme care with positioning. Fragile teeth & veins (difficult IV access)
Patau's syndrome	Trisomy 13 1 in 10,000 live births	Mental retardation, microcephaly, cleft lip/palate, micrognathia. CCD (VSD). Polydactyly Die in infancy	**Possible difficult intubation** Assess cardiac function

COMMON SYNDROMES & CONGENITAL CONDITIONS (7)

Syndrome	Description	Clinical features	Anaesthetic considerations
Pierre Robin syndrome	1 in 8000 live births	Micrognathia, glossoptosis, cleft lip/palate. More severe in neonate (may get airway obstruction) CCD may be present	Improves with growth Assess cardiac function **Intubation may be VERY difficult.** (Consider fibre-optic)
Prader-Willi syndrome	Deletion 15q11 – q13	**Neonate**: Hypotonia & poor feeding **Child**: Hyperactive, uncontrolled eating, mental retardation Cardiovascular failure	Hypoglycaemia risk Difficult IV access. OSA common, may require post-op support Low grade pyrexia or hypothermia also seen
Prune Belly syndrome	Absent abdominal musculature	Poor respiratory function and cough Renal abnormalities	Assess renal function Treat as full stomach Control ventilation, epidural useful post-op
Reye's syndrome	Severe metabolic encephalopathy & fatty change in liver	Abnormal LFTs, deranged clotting Raised ICP if untreated	Largely supportive. Avoid liver-metabolised drugs
Seckel syndrome	Autosomal recessive 'Bird-headed dwarfism'	Mental retardation, microcephaly, dwarfism, micrognathia & prominent maxilla	**Possible difficult ventilation, intubation** and IV access
Sickle cell disease	Abnormal Hb (HbS) which distorts in low O_2 levels (vaso-occlusive crisis or 'Sickling')	**Trait**: (Low HbS levels <50%) Sickling very unlikely **Disease**: (HbS >50%) May present with painful crisis, or sickle peri-op (lung infarction, haemolysis & pain)	Pre-op screening of at-risk groups Crisis: Analgesia (PCA) Peri-op: Avoid prolonged fasting, hydrate well, high FiO_2, keep warm, avoid acidosis. Extreme care with tourniquets
Sleep apnoea	Disorders of breathing during sleep	**Central**: CNS immaturity, trauma, infection or neoplasms. Normal muscle activity **Obstructive**: Obesity, adenotonsillar hyper-trophy or Pierre Robin Response to CO_2 reduced Very sensitive to opiates **Mixed**: Daytime somnolence, snore, insomnia, fatigue, behavioural problems	Review sleep study Careful airway assessment, **intubation may be difficult**. Avoid sedating pre-med Caution with opiates Post-op apnoea monitoring HDU if: < 2 yrs, syndrome affecting airway, CLD for RDS, cor pulmonale
Smith-Lemli-Opitz syndrome	Inborn error of cholesterol synthesis	Microcephaly, mental retardation & hypotonia Skeletal abnormalities, inc. micrognathia	Care with asepsis. Use muscle relaxants with care, **may have airway & intubation problems**

COMMON SYNDROMES & CONGENITAL CONDITIONS (8)

Syndrome	Description	Clinical features	Anaesthetic considerations
Soto's syndrome	Cerebral gigantism	Excessive growth in early childhood Mild developmental delay & macrocephaly Poor immune function Hypotonia	Care with asepsis and positioning of head Hyperthermia has been reported (not MH); monitor temperature
Stickler's syndrome	Autosomal dominant mid-face disorder	Mid-face hypoplasia, micrognathia, cleft palate	Similar to Pierre Robin **Airway may be VERY difficult**
Sturge Weber syndrome	Port-wine stain over Trigeminal nerve distribution	Glaucoma, mental retardation, seizures & hemiplegia	Often multiple laser treatments. May affect larynx
Treacher-Collins syndrome	Mandibulofacial dysplasia	Micrognathia, aplastic zygoma, choanal atresia & cleft lip/palate	Pre-op assessment of cardiac function & airway **May be VERY difficult ventilation/intubation**
Turner's syndrome	XO females	Short stature, infantile genitalia, webbed neck Possible micrognathia CCD (coarctation) Renal anomalies	Assess cardiac & renal status **Intubation may be difficult**
VATER/VACTERL	Non-random association of defects (at least 3)	V – Vertebral (scoliosis) A – Ano-rectal atresia C – Cardiac T – Tracheoesophageal fistula E – oEsophageal atresia R – Renal abnormalities L – Limb defects	Careful pre-op assessment of neonate showing one or more feature Cardiac & renal assessment
Velocardiofacial syndrome	22q11 micro-deletion Very variable presentation	Learning difficulties (mild), small stature. CCD common (VSD, Tetralogy of Fallot). Cleft lip/palate Characteristic facial features	Assess cardiac function **Airway may be difficult**, post-op apnoea monitor essential
Von Recklinghausen's Disease Neurofibromatosis type 1	Café au lait spots (> 5), tumours in all parts of the CNS and peripheral nerves	Very variable. Cutaneous lesions common. May have tumours in larynx or trachea. 50% have kyphoscoliosis. May have fibrosing alveolitis. Renal artery dysplasia common 1% have pheochromocytoma	Assess pulmonary, cardiac & renal function **Intubation my be difficult** Caution with neck Effects of neuromuscular blocking drugs may be prolonged
West's syndrome	Infantile spasms, psychomotor developmental arrest & hypsarrhythmia on EEG	Seizures, neurological deficit & severe mental deficiency	May be difficult to determine level of consciousness. BIS may be unreliable

MANAGEMENT OF ANAPHYLAXIS

Diagnosis & Recognition	Signs and symptoms • **Airway** – Swelling, hoarseness, stridor • **Breathing** – Tachypnoea, wheeze, desaturation • **Circulation** – Pale, clammy, hypotension, tachycardia • **Disability** – Drowsy • **Exposure** – Rash
Immediate management	• **Call for help** • High flow O_2 • Ensure airway secure • Ensure IV access • Lie flat & elevate legs
Treatment	**ADRENALINE** **Intramuscular doses** of 1:1000 • Under 6 years = 150 microgram IM (0.15 mL) • Age 6 – 12 years = 300 microgram IM (0.3 mL) • > 12 years = 500 microgram IM (0.5 mL) Or **Intravenous adrenaline** (1:10,000) • Titrate 1 microgram/kg boluses • Repeat as required at 5 min intervals **IV FLUIDS** • **STOP colloid** - may be the cause! • 20 mL/kg crystalloid bolus

	IV CHLORPHENAMINE	IV HYDROCORTISONE
Child under 6 months	250 microgram/kg	25 mg
6 months to 6 years	2.5 mg	50 mg
6 – 12 years	5 mg	100 mg
> 12 years	10 mg	200 mg

MANAGEMENT AIRWAY EMERGENCIES

Inhaled foreign body • Toddler • Witnessed or unwitnessed acute event • Inspiratory stridor	<u>Anaesthesia for rigid bronchoscopy:</u> D/W ENT surgeon re: plan & check equipment • Slow Gas Induction (sevoflurane in O_2) vs. propofol TCI ➢ Avoid N_2O ➢ Deep laryngoscopy and lignocaine spray to the cords ➢ Maintain spontaneous respiration ➢ 'Short' nasal ET tube to maintain gas delivery while scope being passed • Pass Storz paediatric bronchoscope through the larynx & attach circuit to side arm to maintain anaesthesia • When FB is grasped the forceps & bronchoscope are withdrawn from the trachea as a single unit, SV maintained via face mask or nasopharyngeal airway until the bronchoscope is reintroduced & manoeuvre is repeated as necessary • Monitoring – patient, chest movement, HR & SaO_2. Often lose $EtCO_2$/gas analysis • Possible complications – laryngospasm, bronchospasm, pneumothorax & arrhythmias • **End of procedure** – back to face mask or nasopharyngeal airway & wake up ➢ May benefit from **IV dexamethasone 0.1 – 0.25 mg/kg** for laryngeal oedema ➢ Need continuous SaO_2 monitoring post-op ➢ Consider PHDU or PICU	

Bronchiolitis
 	
• Children < 2 yrs
• Seasonal
• Coryzal symptoms, dry cough, apnoeas, poor feeding
	• Maintenance of oxygenation, with SaO_2 > 92%, using nasal cannula, head box or humidified face mask O_2
	• Small, frequent oral feeds or NG feeds if RR >60/min or oral intake < 50% expected
	• Naso-pharyngeal suction
	• Indications for PHDU/PICU: Recurrent apnoeas
	            Worsening respiratory distress
	            Inability to maintain SaO_2 > 92%
	• PICU management – Intubate and ventilate	

Croup • 6 months – 6 yrs • Barking cough, inspiratory stridor • Symptoms often worse at night • +/- fever	Mild/ moderate	• Dexamethasone : 0.6 mg/kg PO • Budesonide : Nebulised 2 mg (if not tolerating oral medication)
	Severe	• Budesonide : (as above) • Adrenaline < 1 yr: 2.5 mL & 2.5 mL saline (nebulised) >1 yr : 5 mL • **Beware rebound worsening of symptoms** • Dexamethasone : 0.6 mg/kg IV • Transfer to PICU/PHDU – Consider intubation (smaller than expected ET tube)
Epiglottitis • 2 – 7 yr olds • No prodromal illness, toxic • Drooling saliva • Cherry red epiglottis/arytenoids	• **Leave in favoured position, administer oxygen in non-threatening manner** • Call for senior help – Anaesthetist and ENT surgeon Arrange transfer to theatre • Slow Gas Induction with sevoflurane & oxygen ➢ Maintaining spontaneous ventilation in the sitting position ➢ IV access once anaesthetised • Usually requires a smaller than expected ETT • Sedate and ventilate on PICU until a leak appears around the ETT • **IV ceftriaxone or ampicillin**	

MANAGEMENT OF SEPTIC SHOCK

Recognition:
- Fever, tachycardia & abnormal perfusion
- +/- tachypnoea/SpO₂ < 95%, reduced urine output, irritability, lethargy/drowsiness, base deficit on ABG, hypotension (late sign)

COLD Shock
- Capillary refill > 3 sec
- Reduced peripheral pulses
- Cool mottled extremities
- Narrow pulse pressure

WARM shock
- Flash capillary refill
- Bounding peripheral pulses
- Warm extremities
- Wide pulse pressure

IV Antibiotic Therapy
- Child < 28 days
    - **Cefotaxime** 50 mg/kg
    - **Gentamicin** 4 mg/kg (over 3 min)
    - **Amoxicillin** 100 mg/kg
    - Consider **Aciclovir** 20 mg/kg
- Child 28 days – 3 months
    - **Cefotaxime** 50 mg/kg
    - **Gentamicin** 7 mg/kg (over 30 min)
    - **Amoxicillin** 50 mg/kg
- Child > 3 months old
    - **Ceftriaxone** 80 mg/kg (slowly)
    - **Gentamicin** 7 mg/kg (over 30 min)

Coagulopathy
- Treat with: **10 – 20 mL/kg FFP/Octaplas**
- Low fibrinogen suggests DIC : give **5 – 10 mL/kg of Cryoprecipitate**

Dopamine
- To make up (for **CENTRAL** use):
30 mg/kg in 50 mL 5% Dextrose
(1 mL/hr = 10 microgram/kg/min)

High flow O₂ (SaO₂ >95%)
Establish IV or IO access
Check blood sugar

⬇

Initial resuscitation
➤ Bolus 20 mL/kg 0.9% saline or 4.5% HAS until perfusion improves or lung crackles develop (may need > 60 mL/kg)
➤ Correct hypoglycaemia: 2 mL/kg 10% Dextrose
➤ Start antibiotics

⬇

Fluid refractory shock
Call PICU SpR
Start: **Dopamine up to 15 microgram/kg/min IV/IO**
Intubate & gain central access
(Use Ketamine/Fentanyl & Suxamethonium
ETT cuffed if possible, NG tube, urinary catheter)

⬇   ⬇

For Cold Shock   **For Warm Shock**
Add in central Adrenaline   Add in central
if Dopamine resistant   Noradrenaline

⬇

Catecholamine-resistant shock
Start Hydrocortisone (after D/W PICU)

⬇

Transfer to PICU
(Check Ca²⁺, Mg²⁺, K⁺)

Goals of Resuscitation
Restore:-
Normal perfusion, normal HR, BP & RR (for age), normal mental status, UO > 1 mL/kg/hr & serum lactate < 2

MANAGEMENT OF STATUS EPILEPTICUS

- **Confirm clinically that it is an epileptic seizure**:
  - Generalised convulsion lasting ≥ 30 min

  or

  - Repeated convulsions occurring over a 30 min period without recovery of consciousness between convulsions

- **Consider what pre-hospital treatment has been received and modify the protocol accordingly**

- Buccal Midazolam may be given by ambulance crew or parents in non-hospital setting

- If BM < 3.0 mmol/L administer **2 mL/kg 10% Dextrose**

- **Paraldehyde 0.8 mL/kg** of 50:50 paraldehyde/olive oil mixture PR may be administered as directed by senior staff (max 20 mL)

- Inform PICU & Anaesthetic Teams when considering loading with **Phenytoin**

- **Phenytoin** administration
  - Doses <500 mg in 50 mL
  - Doses >500 mg in 250 mL

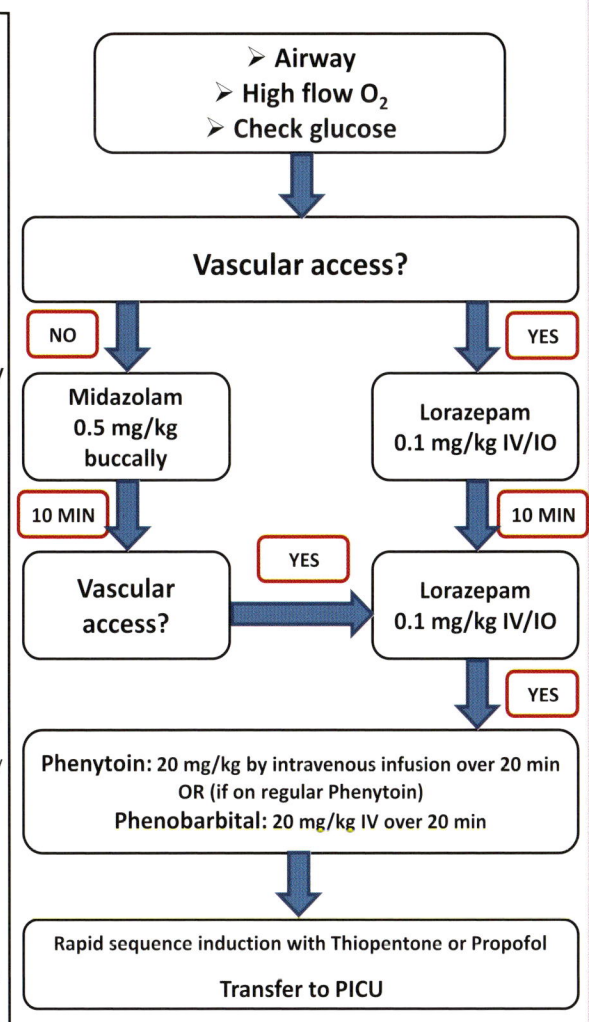

- Airway
- High flow O$_2$
- Check glucose

Vascular access?

NO → Midazolam 0.5 mg/kg buccally
YES → Lorazepam 0.1 mg/kg IV/IO

10 MIN

Vascular access? → YES → Lorazepam 0.1 mg/kg IV/IO

10 MIN

YES

Phenytoin: 20 mg/kg by intravenous infusion over 20 min
OR (if on regular Phenytoin)
Phenobarbital: 20 mg/kg IV over 20 min

Rapid sequence induction with Thiopentone or Propofol

Transfer to PICU

MANAGEMENT OF ACUTE LIFE-THREATENING ASTHMA

Diagnosis & Recognition	- Reduced consciousness/agitated - Silent chest - Fatigue, exhaustion - Poor respiratory effort - Cyanosis in air (SaO_2 < 92% in air) - PEFR < 33% expected
Immediate management	- High flow O_2 to keep SpO_2 > 92% - Get senior help (Paeds SpR/Anaes SpR/PICU) - Establish IV or IO access - Monitoring: ECG & SpO_2

Treatment	**NEBULISERS**
	- Back-to-back **salbutamol** nebs (O_2 driven)
	    – 2.5 mg under 5 years **OR** 5 mg over 5 years
	- **Ipratropium** nebs (250 microgram) every 20 min in 1st hour
	INTRAVENOUS INFUSIONS
	- **Salbutamol I.V.** – Load over 5 min with:
	    - 5 microgram/kg if under 2 yr
	          OR
	    - 15 microgram/kg if over 2 yr (max 250 microgram)
	- **Aminophylline I.V.** – Load with 5 mg/kg over 20 min then 1 mg/kg/hr
	- **Magnesium I.V.** – 0.2 mmol/kg over 20 min
	- **Steroids** – Hydrocortisone 4 mg/kg (max 100 mg)
	- **Crystalloid fluid boluses**

INTUBATION **AVOID IF AT ALL POSSIBLE**	**Indications:** - Cardiac or respiratory arrest - Severe hypoxia - Deteriorating mental state - Progressive exhaustion **CLINICAL JUDGEMENT RATHER THAN BLOOD GASES**	**Considerations:** - Senior help - Consider **RSI with ketamine & suxamethonium** - Lignocaine spray to cords - **Cuffed ETT if possible** - Aim Vt 6 – 8 mL/kg - Avoid PEEP - Long expiratory times - Permissive hypercapnia - Consider paralysis

MANAGEMENT OF DIABETIC KETOACIDOSIS

Diagnosis	**History** - Polyuria, polydipsia, weight loss, abdominal pain, tiredness, vomiting, confusion
	Signs - Dehydration, kussmaul breathing, lethargy/drowsiness
	Biochemical - Blood glucose >11 mmol/L, pH <7.3 or bicarbonate <15 mmol/L, ketouria
Immediate management	<ul><li>**Airway & breathing** - high flow oxygen</li><li>**Circulation** - if shocked, give 10 mL/kg 0.9% sodium chloride, repeat up to 3 times</li><li>**Assess degree of dehydration**<ul><li>Mild (3%) – only just clinically detectable</li><li>Moderate (5%) – dry mucous membranes, reduced skin turgor</li><li>Severe (8%) – above plus sunken eyes, poor capillary return</li></ul></li><li>1% dehydration = 10 mL/kg deficit to be replaced over 48 hr</li><li>Start IV fluid replacement with 0.9% saline and 20 mmol KCl in 500 mL bag</li></ul>

Monitoring & Investigation	<ul><li>Weigh (12 hourly)</li><li>Continuous ECG monitoring</li><li>Hourly BP & urine output</li><li>Hourly GCS until pH > 7.3</li><li>Glucose ½ hourly for first 2 hr, then hourly until 4 – 14 mmol/L, then 2 – 4 hourly thereafter</li><li>Na$^+$, K$^+$ & ABG at 0, 2 & 6 hours</li><li>Capillary blood glucose & ketones every 1 – 2 hr</li></ul>	<ul><li>Glucose, HbA1c</li><li>U&Es</li><li>Venous blood gas</li><li>Serum osmolality</li><li>Urine/blood ketones</li><li>FBC</li><li>LFT</li><li>Amylase</li></ul>

Fluid management	Calculate total volume requirement and plan to replace over 48 hours
	Include: - Deficit – measured or assessed weight loss (1 kg = 1000 mL)
	         - Maintenance requirements
	         - Continuing losses – replaced only if urine output or vomiting is excessive
	Subtract: - Any volume already received during resuscitation
	Hourly rate = $\frac{(48 \text{ hr maintenance + deficit}) - \text{resuscitation fluid already given}}{48}$

Insulin infusion	**Commence insulin infusion an hour after starting IV fluids** (50 units human soluble insulin (Actrapid or Humulin S) per 50 mL 0.9% saline) **Infuse at rate of 0.1 units/kg/hour. An initial bolus should NOT be given** Aim for a gradual fall in glucose of ≈ 5 mmol/L/hr until it reaches 14 mmol/L. If the rate of fall is > 5 mmol/L/hr, add glucose to the IV fluids **If despite increased glucose (up to 10%), blood sugar continues to fall rapidly or is < 4 mmol/L decrease insulin rate to 0.05 units/kg/hr** **DO NOT STOP INSULIN INFUSION** For BM < 4 give a bolus of 2 mL/kg of 10% glucose IV and add extra glucose to the IV fluids, rather than reducing/stopping the insulin If pH > 7.3 with stable blood sugars between 4 – 15 & receiving glucose containing IV fluids, insulin infusion can be reduced to **0.05 units/kg/hr**

MANAGEMENT OF CEREBRAL OEDEMA ASSOCIATED WITH DIABETIC KETOACIDOSIS

Diagnosis	- Up to 1% of children with DKA develop cerebral oedema with a high morbidity/mortality
- Signs – Headache, confusion, irritability or restlessness, reduced conscious level, fits, increasing BP, slowing pulse, papilloedema, abnormal posturing
- Risk appears to be increased if insulin is started within an hour of starting IV fluids. Hence current recommendation to defer the insulin infusion for at least 1 hour after starting fluids
- If cerebral oedema is suspected inform the Paediatric Consultant and PICU team
Emergency management	- Exclude hypoglycaemia and continue insulin infusion
- Give hypertonic saline (2.7%) 5 mL/kg over 5 – 10 min or mannitol 1 g/kg stat (5 mL/kg 20% mannitol in 20 min) as soon as possible
- Restrict IV fluids to ½ maintenance and plan to replace over 72 hours rather than 48 hours
- Continue management on PICU if not already there
- Intubate and ventilate to low normal pCO_2 (4 kPa)
- Exclude other diagnoses by CT scan (thrombosis, infarction or haemorrhage)
- Consider intracranial pressure monitoring
- Repeated doses of mannitol (above dose 2 hourly) may be needed to control intracranial pressure
- Close management of sodium is essential. If outside of the range 140 – 150 mmol/L, discuss with paediatric endocrinologist on-call. Assess the degree of dehydration

FORMULARY (1)

DRUG	INDICATION	DOSE
Acyclovir	Severe sepsis in under 28 day old	20 mg/kg
Adenosine	Management of SVT	100 – 500 microgram/kg (max 12 mg)
Adrenaline	Cardiac arrest Anaphylaxis Croup/airway compromise Low cardiac output - (0.3 mg/kg in 50 mL 5% Dextrose)	IV: 10 microgram/kg IM: 10 microgram/kg Nebulised: 400 microgram/kg Infusion: 0.01 – 1 microgram/kg/min
Alfentanil	Short-term analgesia/Induction	10 microgram/kg
Aminophylline	Life-threatening asthma	5 mg/kg Then: 1 mg/kg/hr
Amiodarone	Arrhythmia management	5 mg/kg (max 1.2 g in 24 hr) Infusion: 300 microgram/kg/hr
Amoxicillin	Severe sepsis	50 – 100 mg/kg
Atracurium	Neuromuscular blockade	0.5 mg/kg Infusion: 0.3 – 0.6 mg/kg/hr
Atropine	Bradycardia Pre-medication (1 hr pre-procedure)	20 microgram/kg (100 – 600 microgram) 30 microgram/kg PO (max 900)
Benzyl-penicillin	Early sepsis in neonates	50 mg/kg
Blood (Packed Red Cells)	Haemorrhage/low Hb (< 80 g/L)	10 – 20 mL/kg (5 mL/kg will ↑ Hb by ~10 g/L)
Bupivacaine (levo-)	Local anaesthetic	2 mg/kg
Calcium Chloride 10%	Hypocalcaemia/Hyperkalaemia	0.2 mL/kg
Calcium Gluconate	Hypocalcaemia-induced cardiac arrest Hyperkalaemia	0.3 mL/kg 10% solution (max 20 mL) 0.5 mL/kg 10% solution (max 20 mL)
Calcium Resonium	Hyperkalaemia	1 g/kg
Cefotaxime	Severe sepsis	50 mg/kg
Ceftriaxone	Severe sepsis	80 mg/kg
Cefuroxime	Surgical prophylaxis	30 – 50 mg/kg
Clonidine	Pre-medication (1 hr pre-procedure)	4 microgram/kg PO 2 microgram/kg Intranasal
Co-Amoxiclav	Surgical prophylaxis	30 mg/kg
Codeine	Analgesia (**over 12 yrs only**)	1 mg/kg/hr (max 60 mg)
Cryoprecipitate	Low fibrinogen (< 1.5 g/L)	5 – 10 mL/kg
Dantrolene	Malignant hyperthermia	2.5 mg/kg Then: 1 mg/kg boluses

FORMULARY (2)

DRUG	INDICATION	DOSE
Dexamethasone	Anti-emetic	0.15 mg/kg
Dextrose 10%	Hypoglycaemia Hyperkalaemia (*with Insulin*)	2 mL/kg 　Then: 5 mL/kg/hr 5 mL/kg/hr
Diazepam	Muscle spasm	0.1 mg/kg QDS
Diclofenac	Analgesia (> 6 months old)	1 mg/kg
Dobutamine	Low cardiac output states - 30 mg/kg in 50 mL 5% Dextrose	5 – 15 microgram/kg/min
Dopamine	Severe sepsis with low cardiac output - 30 mg/kg in 50 mL 5% Dextrose (central) - 3 mg/kg in 50 mL 5% Dextrose (peripheral)	5 – 15 microgram/kg/min
Esmolol	Treatment of arrhythmias	500 microgram/kg over 1 min 　Then: 50 microgram/kg/min over 4 min
Fentanyl	Analgesia/Induction of anaesthesia	1 – 2 microgram/kg
FFP/Octaplas	Coagulopathy/Massive transfusion	10 – 20 mL/kg
Flecanide	Resistant re-entry SVT, VEs or VT	2 mg/kg (max 150 mg)
Flucloxacillin	Surgical prophylaxis	25 mg/kg
Flumazanil	Reversal of benzodiazepine	10 microgram/kg (max 200)
Furosemide	Diuretic	1 – 2 mg/kg
Gentamicin	Surgical prophylaxis Severe sepsis	2 mg/kg 5 – 7 mg/kg
Glycopyrolate	Bradycardia Reversal of neuromuscular blockade	10 microgram/kg
Hydrocortisone	2nd line anaphylaxis	4 mg/kg
	Steroid Replacement Therapy: (if > 10 mg prednisolone (or equivalent) per day) - **Minor** surgery (e.g. hernia repair)	Routine pre-op steroid dose 　OR 1 – 2 mg/kg IV at induction
	- **Intermediate** surgery (e.g. laparoscopic)	Normal dose AND 1 – 2 mg/kg IV at induction & 6 hourly for 24 hr
	- **Major** Surgery (e.g. laparotomy)	Normal dose AND 1 – 2 mg/kg IV at induction & 6 hourly for 48 – 72 hr
	If steroids stopped > 3 months ago – no replacement needed	

FORMULARY (3)

DRUG	INDICATION	DOSE
Ibuprofen	Analgesia (>5 kg)	5 mg/kg
Insulin	Diabetic management Hyperkalaemia (*with 10% Dextrose*)	0.05 – 0.1 units/kg/hr
Intralipid 20%	Local anaesthetic toxicity	1.5 mL/kg; Then: 15 – 30 mL/kg/hr
Ipratropium	Asthma	Nebulised: 250 microgram
Ketamine	Pre-medication (30 min pre-procedure) Induction of anaesthesia	6 mg/kg PO (3 mg/kg if given with midazolam) 1 – 2 mg/kg IM: 5 – 10 mg/kg
Lidocaine	2nd line VF or pulseless VT	1 mg/kg (max 100 mg)
Lorazepam	Pre-medication (1 hr pre-procedure) Status epilepticus	50 – 100 microgram/kg (max 4 mg) 0.1 mg/kg
Magnesium Sulphate	Severe asthma/Torsades de pointes	0.1 – 0.2 mmol/kg (max 8 mmol)
Mannitol 20%	Raised ICP	0.25 – 1 g/kg (0.5 g/kg = 2.5 mL/kg)
Methyl-prednisolone	Renal transplant	300 mg/m^2 over 10 min (max 500 mg)
Metronidazole	Surgical prophylaxis	30 mg/kg
Midazolam	Pre-medication (30 min pre-procedure) Status epilepticus Sedation (*6 mg/kg in 50 mL*)	0.5 mg/kg PO (max 20 mg) 0.3 mg/kg buccal (max 5mg) Buccal: 0.5 mg/kg Infusion: 60 – 240 microgram/kg/hr
Morphine	Analgesia: - Low dose (codeine replacement) Sedation (*1 mg/kg in 50 mL*)	IV: 0.1 mg/kg Oral: 0.1 – 0.5 mg/kg < 1 yr: 50 – 100 microgram/kg PO > 1 yr: 100 – 200 microgram/kg PO Infusion: 10 – 40 microgram/kg/hr
Naloxone	Reversal of opiates	10 microgram/kg Infusion: 5 – 20 microgram/kg/hr
Neostigmine	Reversal of neuromuscular blockade	50 microgram/kg
Noradrenaline	Acute hypotension - 0.3 mg/kg in 50 mL 5% Dextrose	Infusion: 0.01 – 0.5 microgram/kg/min
Ondansetron	Anti-emetic/Opiate-induced pruritus	0.15 mg/kg
Paracetamol	Analgesia	Oral: 15 – 20 mg/kg IV: - Prem > 32 weeks – 7.5 mg/kg TDS - Neonate – 10 mg/kg QDS - Child < 50 kg – 15 mg/kg QDS
Paraldehyde	Status epilepticus	PR: 0.8 mL/kg (max 20 mL)

FORMULARY (4)

DRUG	INDICATION	DOSE
Phenobarbital	Status epilepticus	20 mg/kg over 20 min
Phenylephrine	Acute hypotension	1 microgram/kg
Phenytoin	Status epilepticus	20 mg/kg over 20 min
Piperacillin (with Tazobactam)	Septicaemia	90 mg/kg (max 4.5 g)
Piriton	2nd line anaphylaxis/Pruritus	0.1 mg/kg (max 4 mg PO, or 5 mg IV)
Platelets	Low platelets (< 75 x 10^9/L)	10 – 20 mL/kg
Propofol	Induction of anaesthesia Maintenance of anaesthesia	1 – 4 mg/kg Infusion: 4 – 12 mg/kg/hr
Prostin	Opening/maintaining PDA in neonate	5 nanogram/kg/min (max 100 nanogram/kg/min)
Rocuronium	Neuromuscular blockade	1 mg/kg Infusion: 0.3 – 1 mg/kg/hr
Salbutamol	Asthma	Nebulised: 2.5 – 10 mg IV: 5 microgram/kg (Under 2 yr) 15 microgram/kg (Over 2 yr)
Saline 2.7%	Raised intra cranial pressure	5 mL/kg
Sodium Bicarbonate	Metabolic acidosis/Hyperkalaemia	0.5 – 1 mL/kg of 8.4% solution
Sugammadex	Reversal of Rocuronium – Routine Immediate	2 – 4 mg/kg 16 mg/kg
Suxamethonium	Neuromuscular blockade	1 – 2 mg/kg
Teicoplanin	Surgical prophylaxis	10 mg/kg over 30 min
Temazepam	Pre-medication (1 hr pre-procedure) (Age: 12 – 18 yr)	10 – 20 mg/kg
Thiopentone	Induction of anaesthesia	3 – 5 mg/kg
Tranexamic Acid	Massive haemorrhage	15 mg/kg Then: 2 mg/kg/hr
Vancomycin	Surgical prophylaxis	15 mg/kg over 60 min
Vecuronium	Neuromuscular blockade	0.1 mg/kg Infusion: 0.8 – 1.4 microgram/kg/hr

NOTES

References

- Weight information:
  - 1 – 12 months = (0.5 x age in months) + 4
  - 1 – 5 years = (2 x age) + 8
  - 6 – 12 years = (3 x age) + 7
  - UK – WHO growth charts – www.rcpch.ac.uk/growthcharts
- BNF for Children 2013 – 2014
- Advanced Paediatric Life Support. The Practical Approach. 5th Edition
- Association of Anaesthetists of Great Britain and Ireland. Blood transfusion and the anaesthetist: Management of massive haemorrhage. *Anaesthesia* 2010; **65**: 1153-1161
- Major trauma and the use of tranexamic acid in children, RCPCH, November 2012
- Head injury: triage, assessment, investigation and early management of head injury in infants, children and adults NICE Clinical Guideline 176, January 2014. www.nice.org.uk/guidance/CG176
- "Emergency Management of Severe Burns", course manual. Australian and New Zealand Burn Association/UK version for the British Burn Association, 15th Edition, June 2012
- Paediatric Airway Guidelines 2012 – The Guidelines Group, supported by the Association of Paediatric Anaesthetists, the Difficult Airway Society and liaising with the RCoA. Reproduced with permission
- Malignant Hyperthermia Crisis – AAGBI Safety Guideline 2013
- Management of severe local anaesthetic toxicity 2 – AAGBI Safety Guideline 2010
- Good Practice in Postoperative and Procedural Pain Management, 2nd Edition. APAGBI, July 2012
- APA consensus guideline on peri-operative fluid management in children v 1.1, September 2007
- Resuscitation Council (UK) Emergency treatment of anaphylactic reactions. January 2008, annotated July 2012
- Bacterial meningitis and meningococcal septicaemia. NICE Clinical Guideline 102, June 2010. www.nice.org.uk/guidance/CG102
- Management of status epilepticus NICE Clinical Guidelines CG137 (published 2011) . www.nice.org.uk/guidance/CG137
- British Guideline on the Management of Asthma. SIGN & The British Thoracic Society, revised May 2011
- DKA guidelines. British Society of Paediatric Endocrinology and Diabetes website. www.bsped.org.uk